# STICKY BACKEY

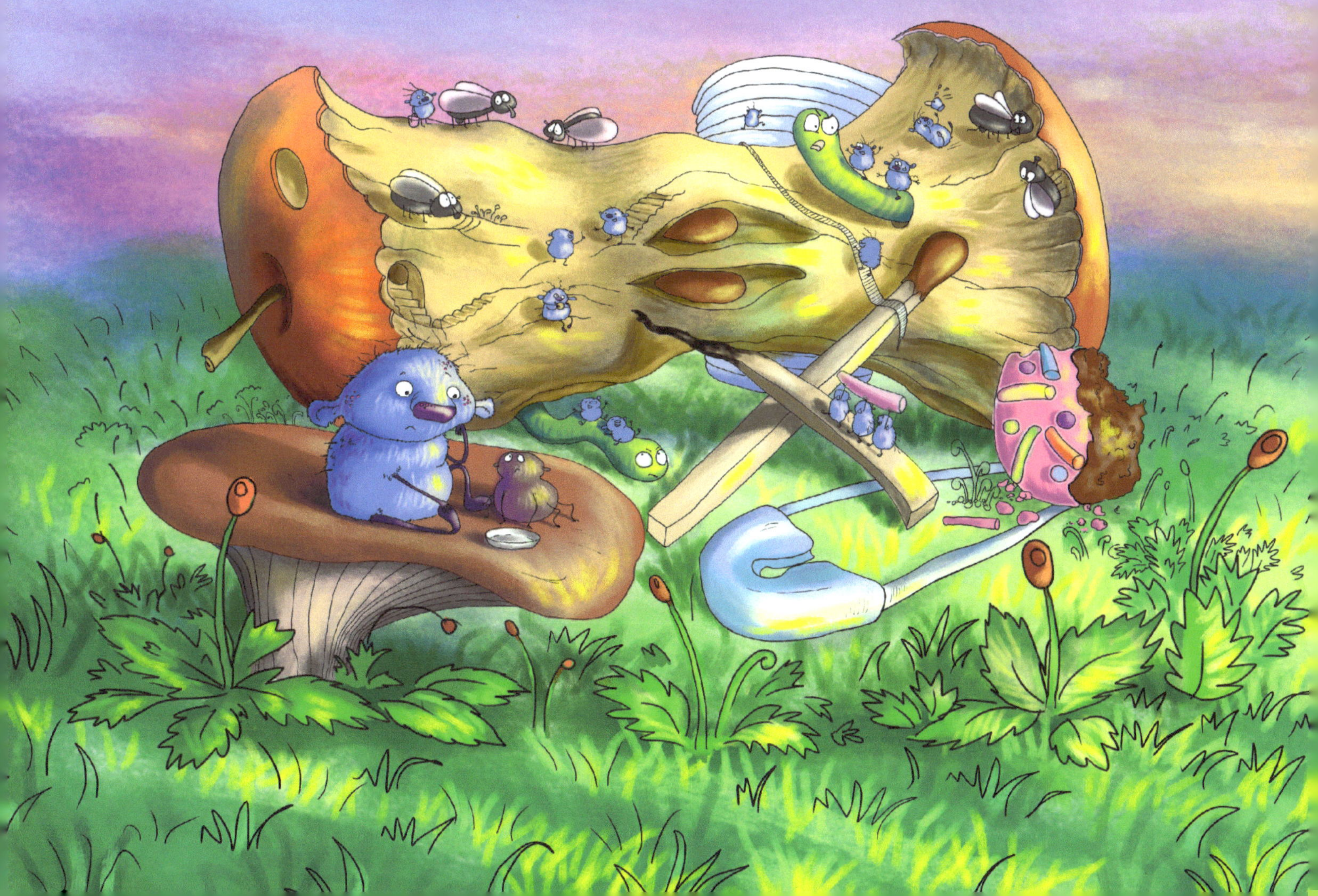

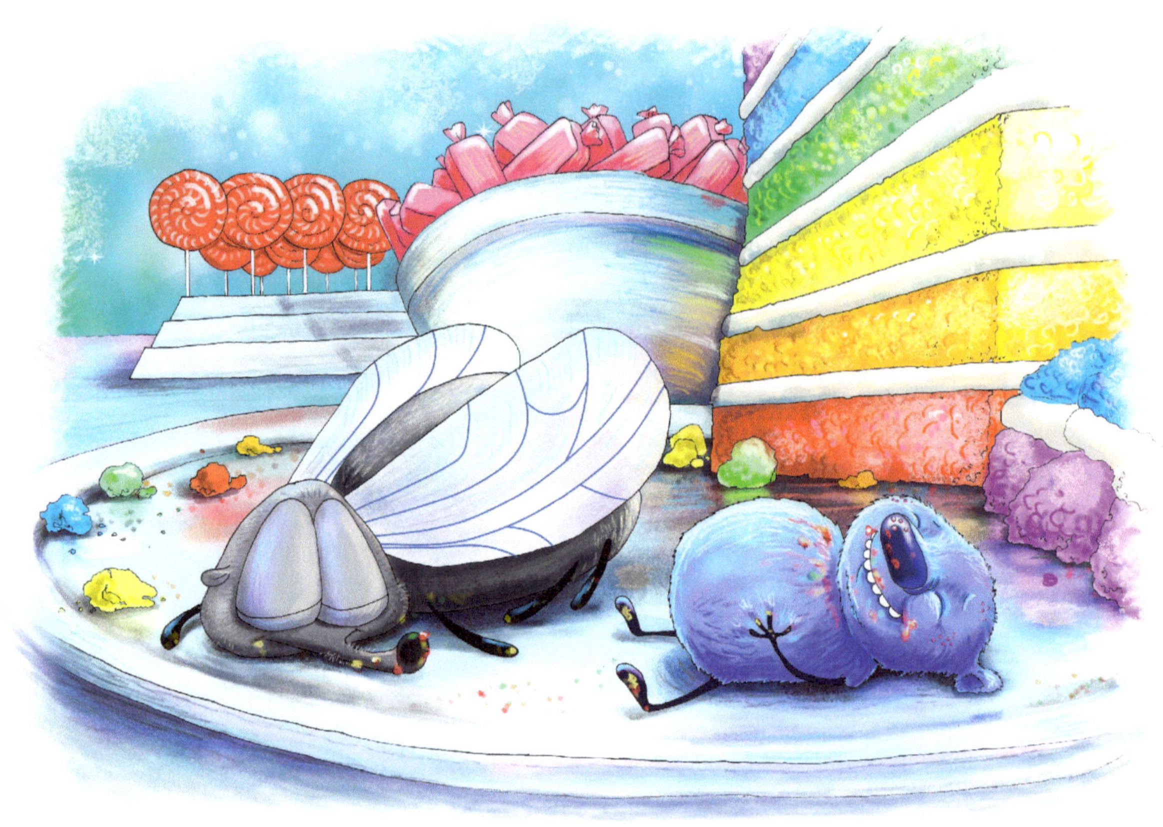

Text and illustrations copyright © 2022 Viktoriia Oliinyk



ISBN: 979-8-8330-2243-6

vikty@live.com

# STICKY BACKEY

## Written and illustrated by
## Viktoriia Oliinyk

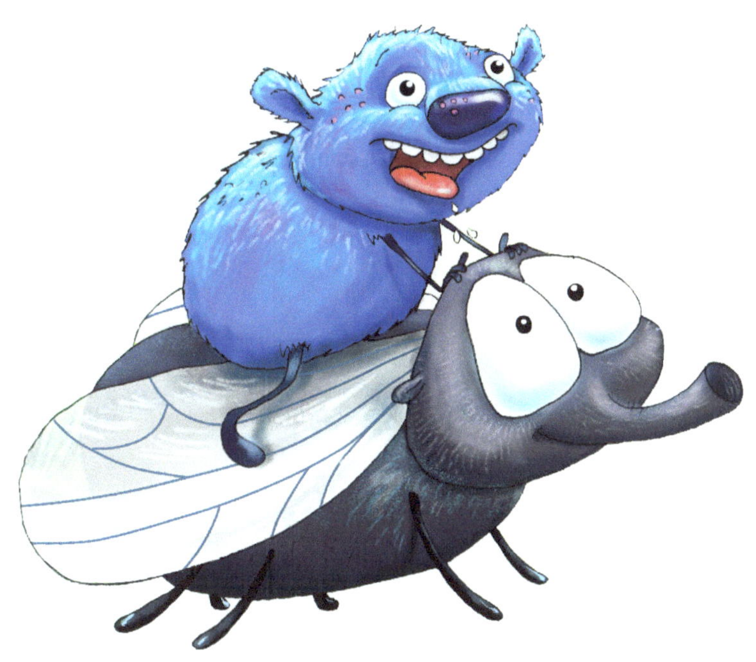

Edited by
Emily Abdelmegid

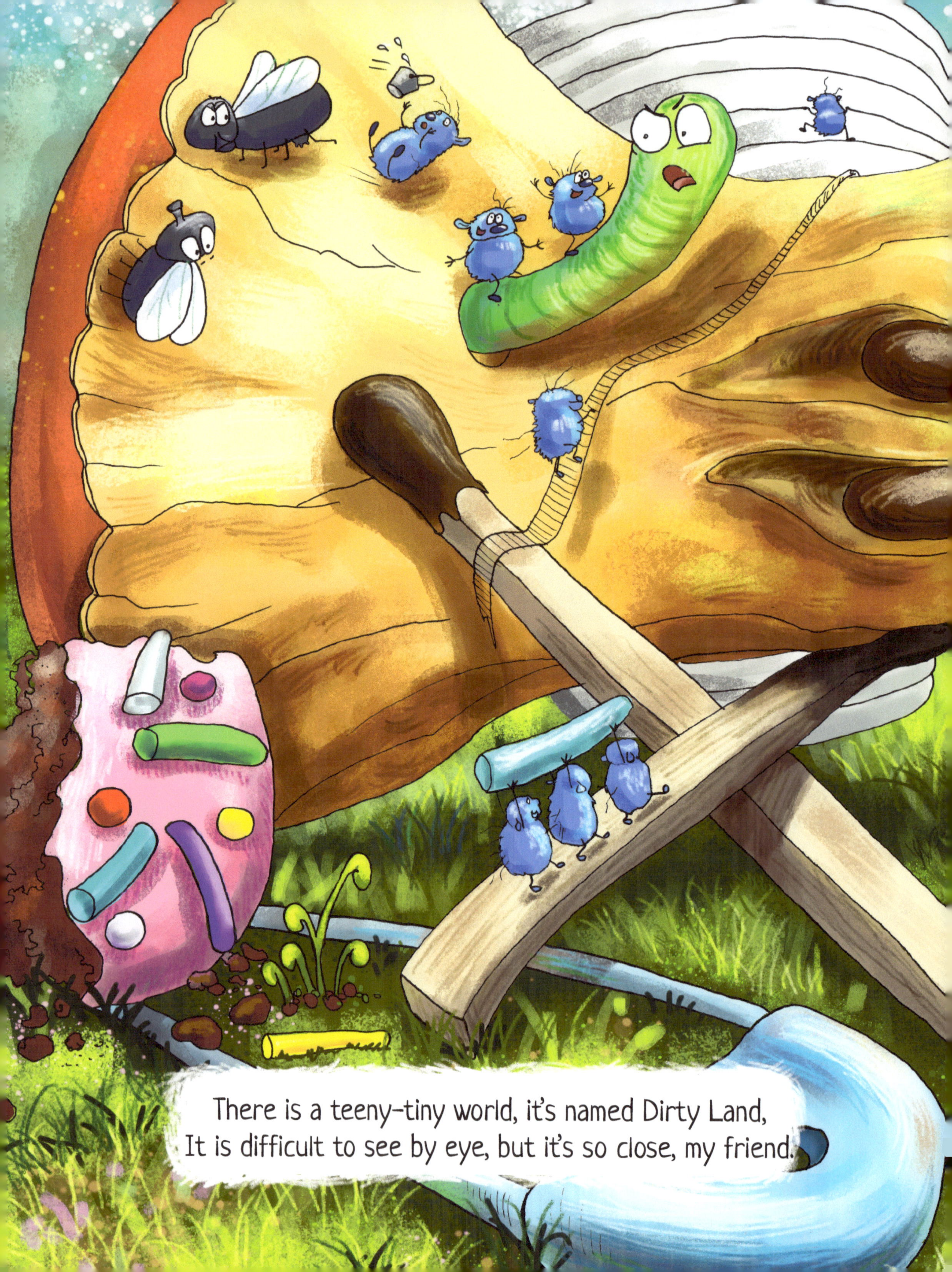

There is a teeny-tiny world, it's named Dirty Land,
It is difficult to see by eye, but it's so close, my friend.

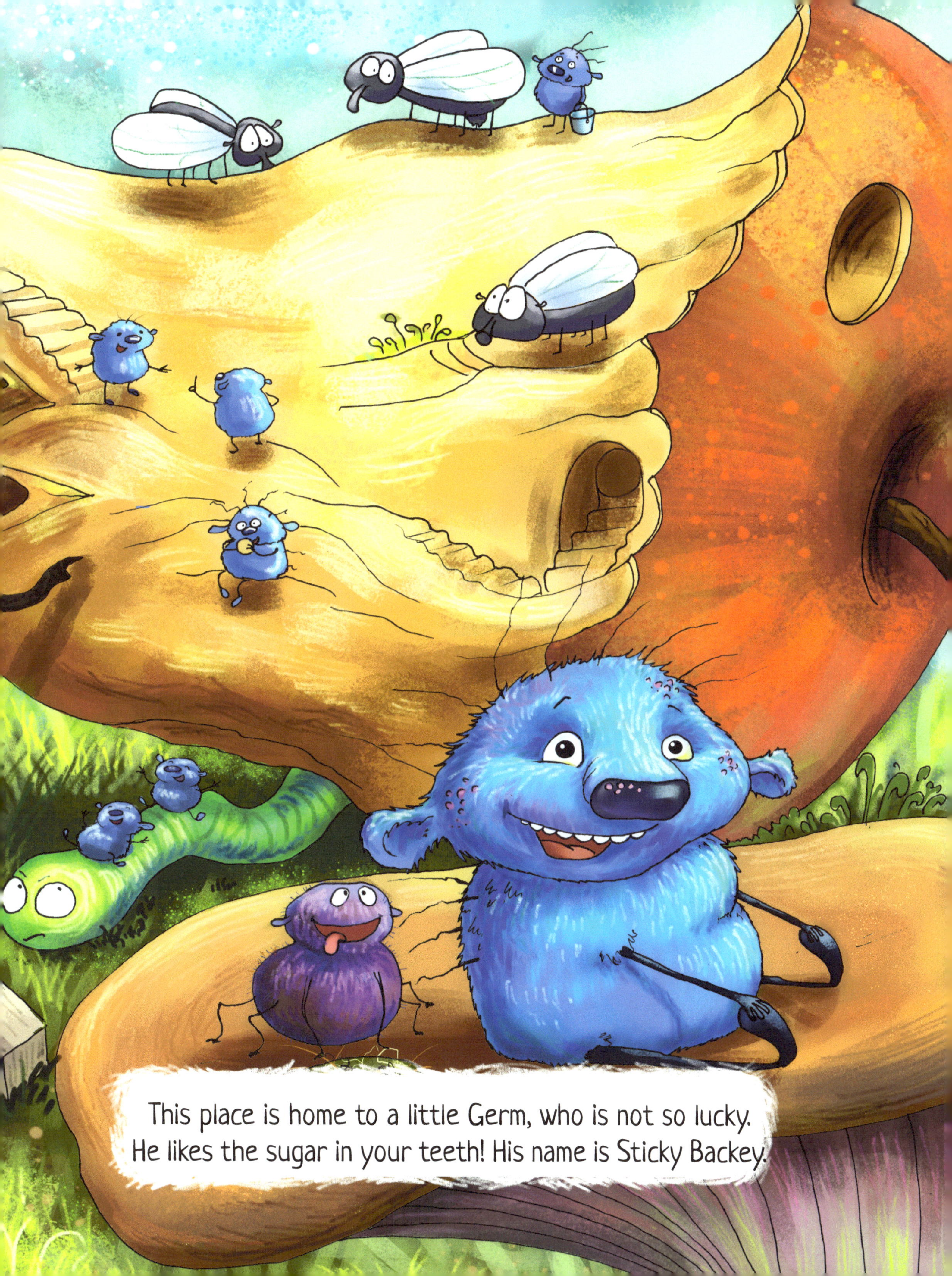

This place is home to a little Germ, who is not so lucky.
He likes the sugar in your teeth! His name is Sticky Backey.

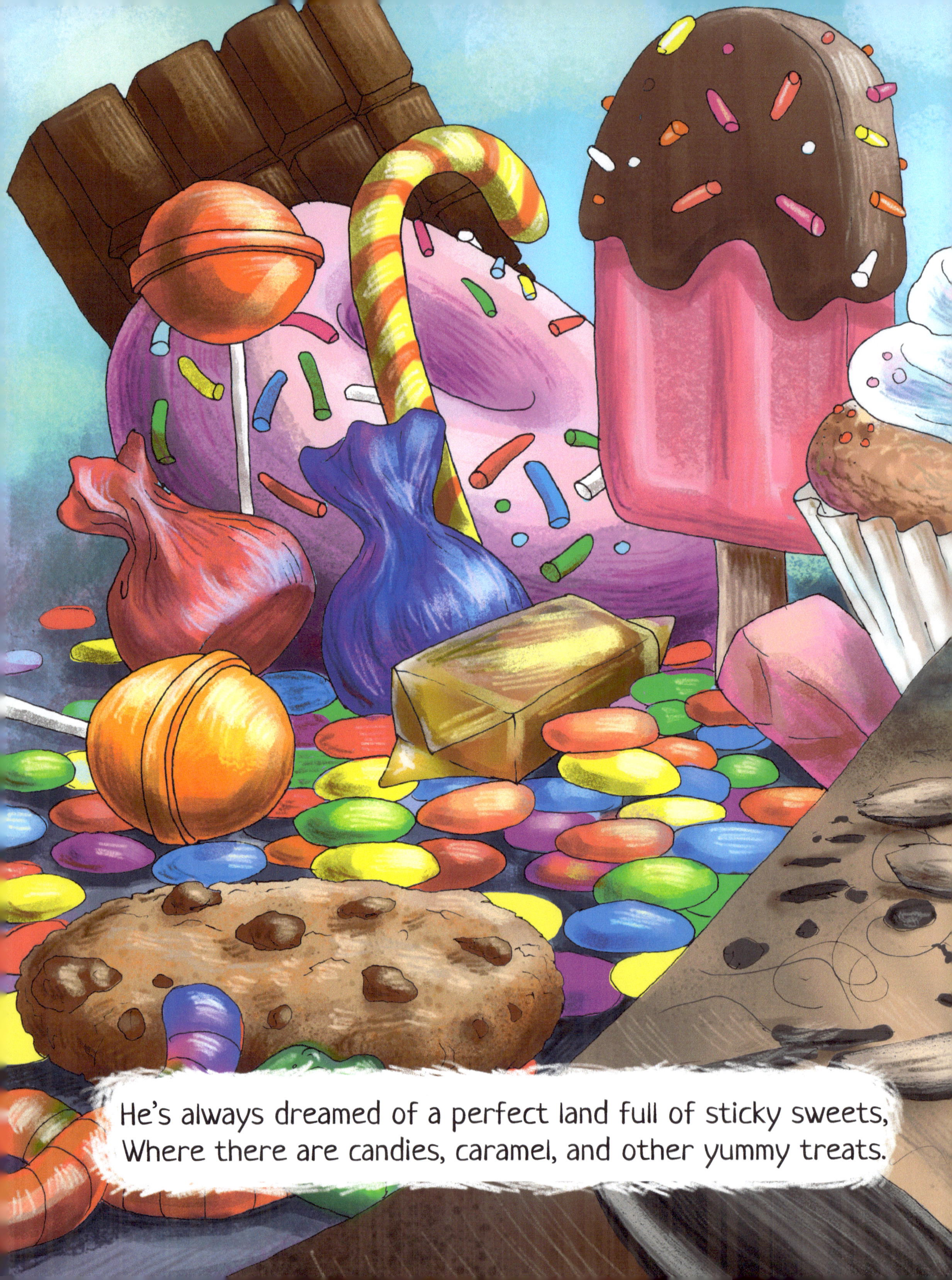

He's always dreamed of a perfect land full of sticky sweets,
Where there are candies, caramel, and other yummy treats.

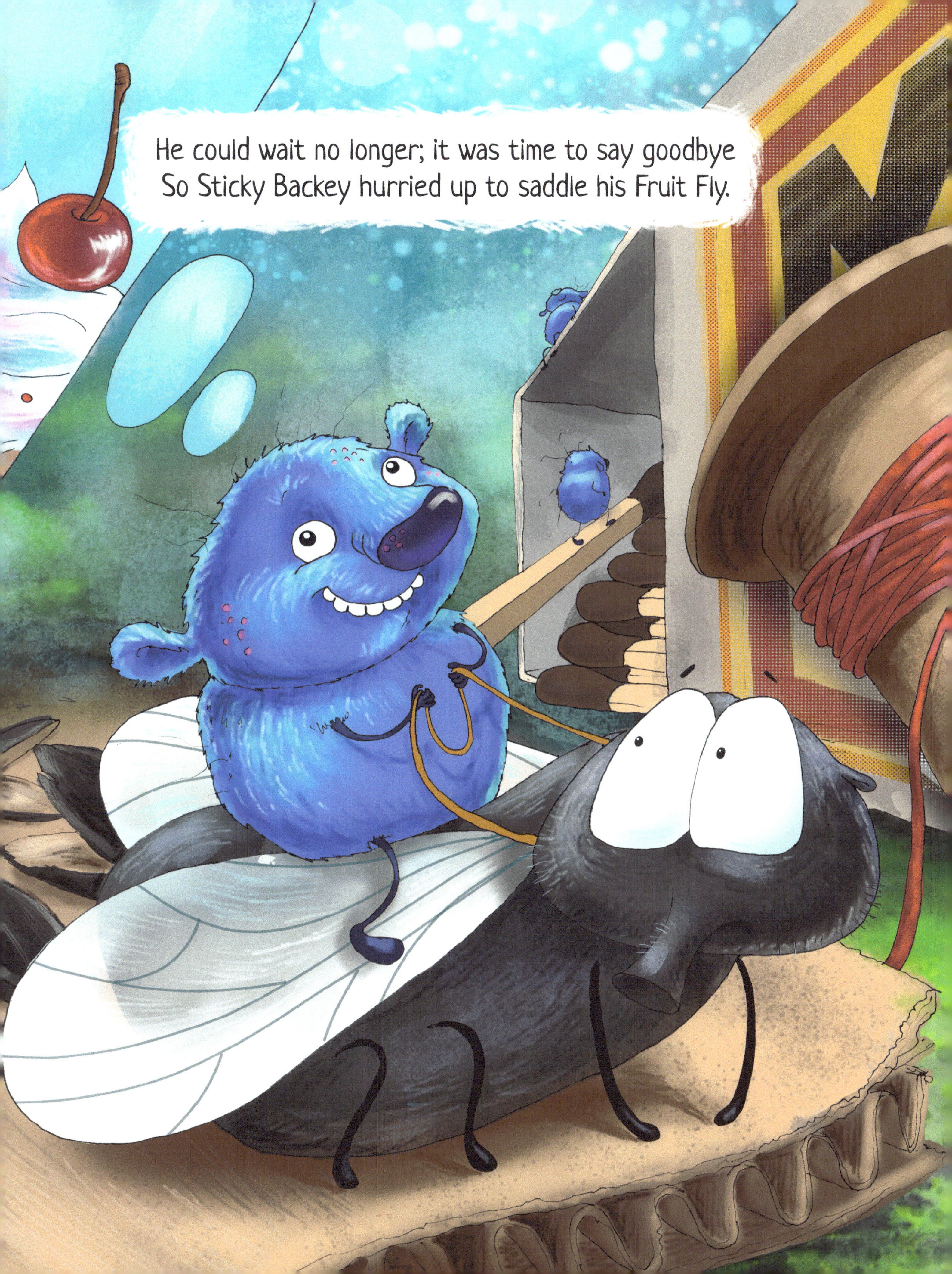

He could wait no longer; it was time to say goodbye
So Sticky Backey hurried up to saddle his Fruit Fly.

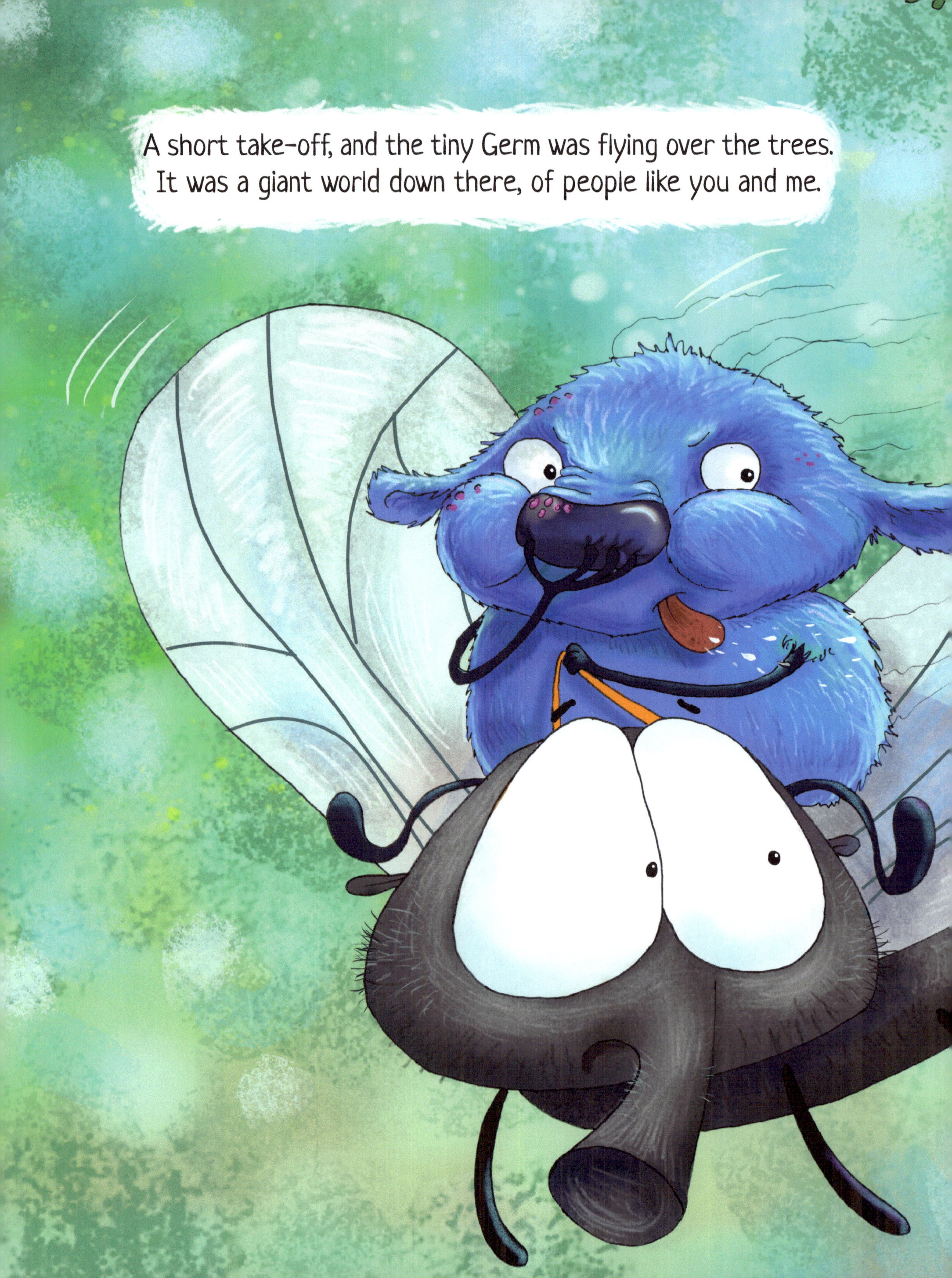
A short take-off, and the tiny Germ was flying over the trees.
It was a giant world down there, of people like you and me.

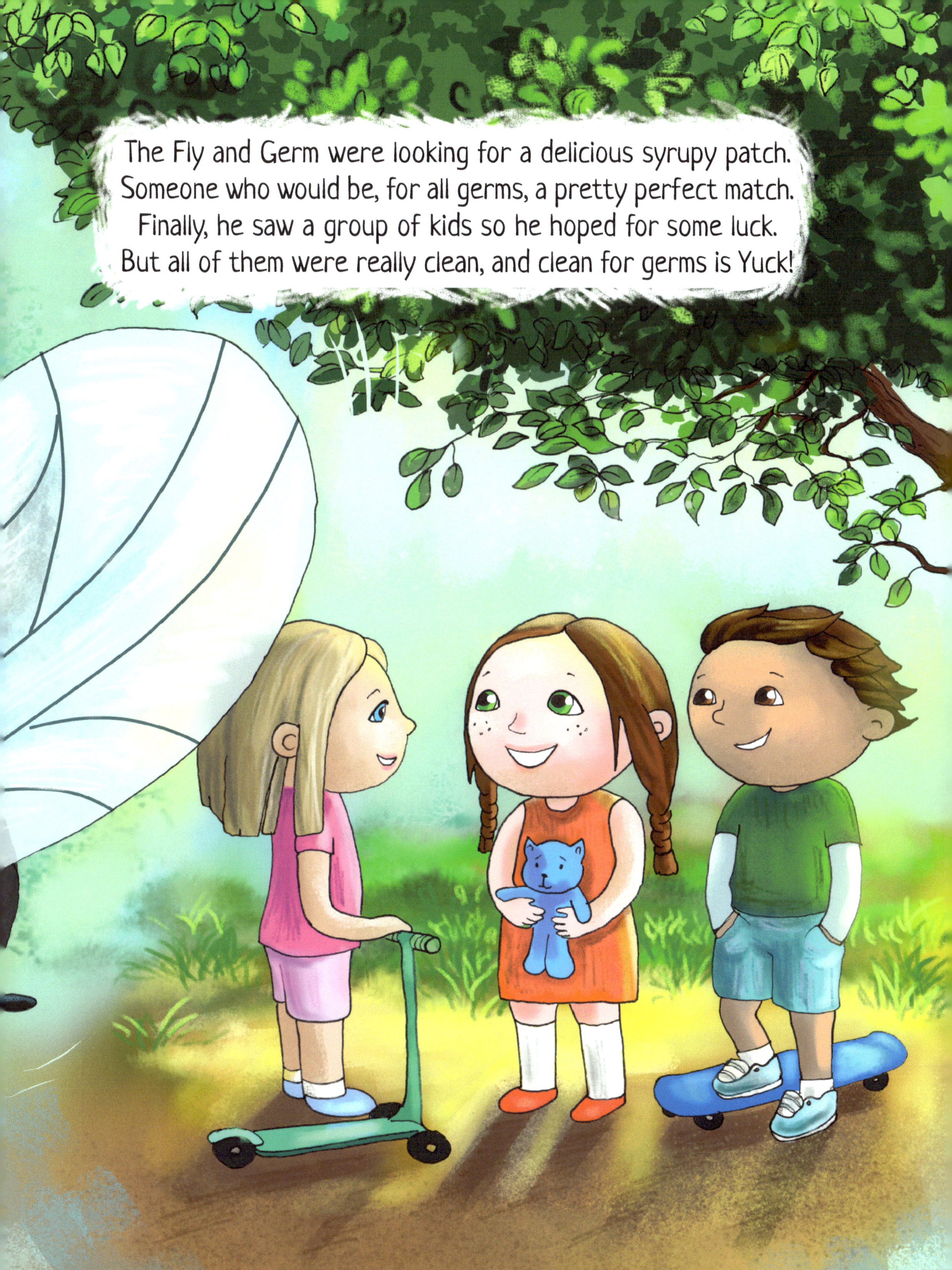

The Fly and Germ were looking for a delicious syrupy patch.
Someone who would be, for all germs, a pretty perfect match.
Finally, he saw a group of kids so he hoped for some luck.
But all of them were really clean, and clean for germs is Yuck!

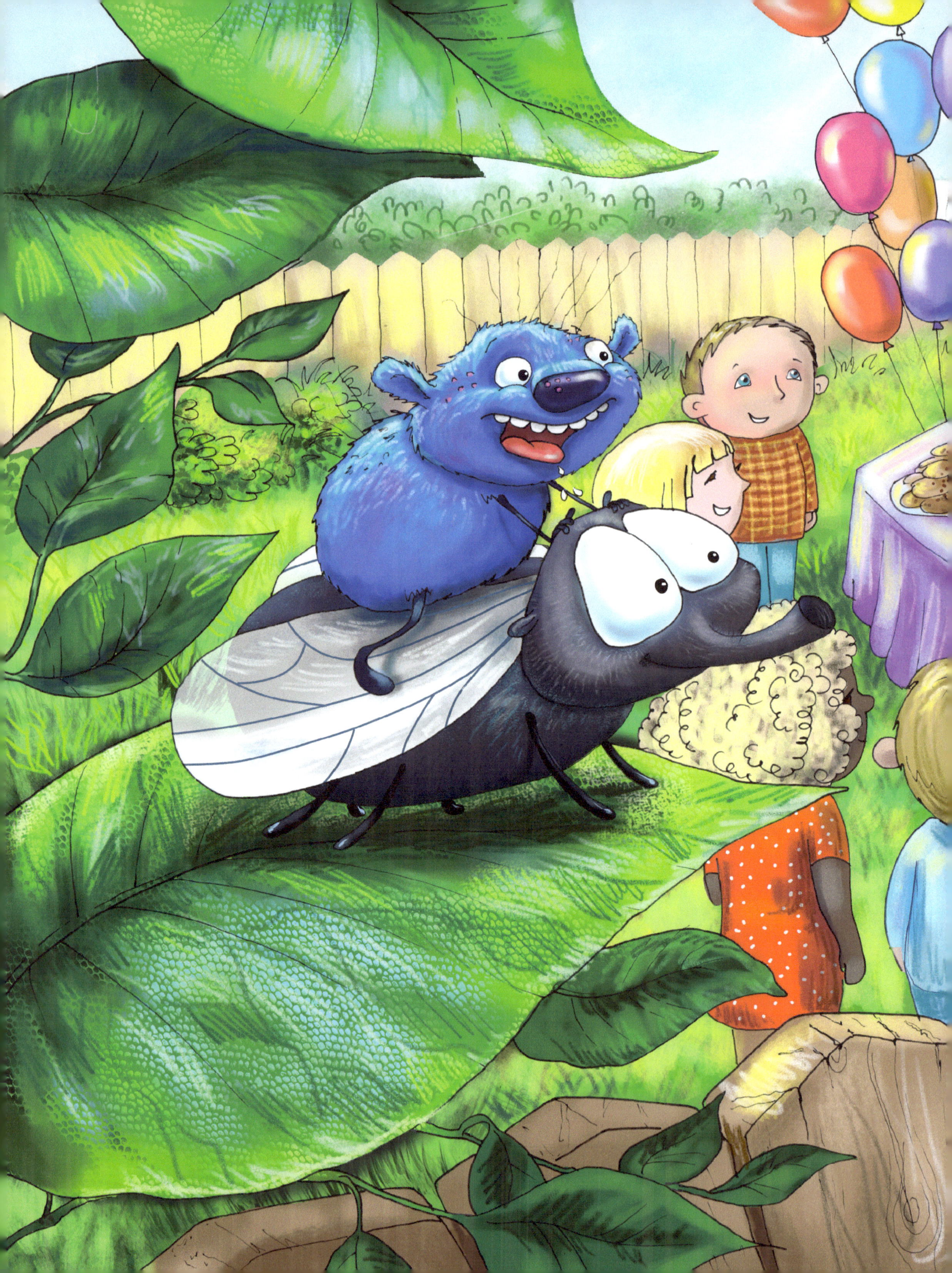

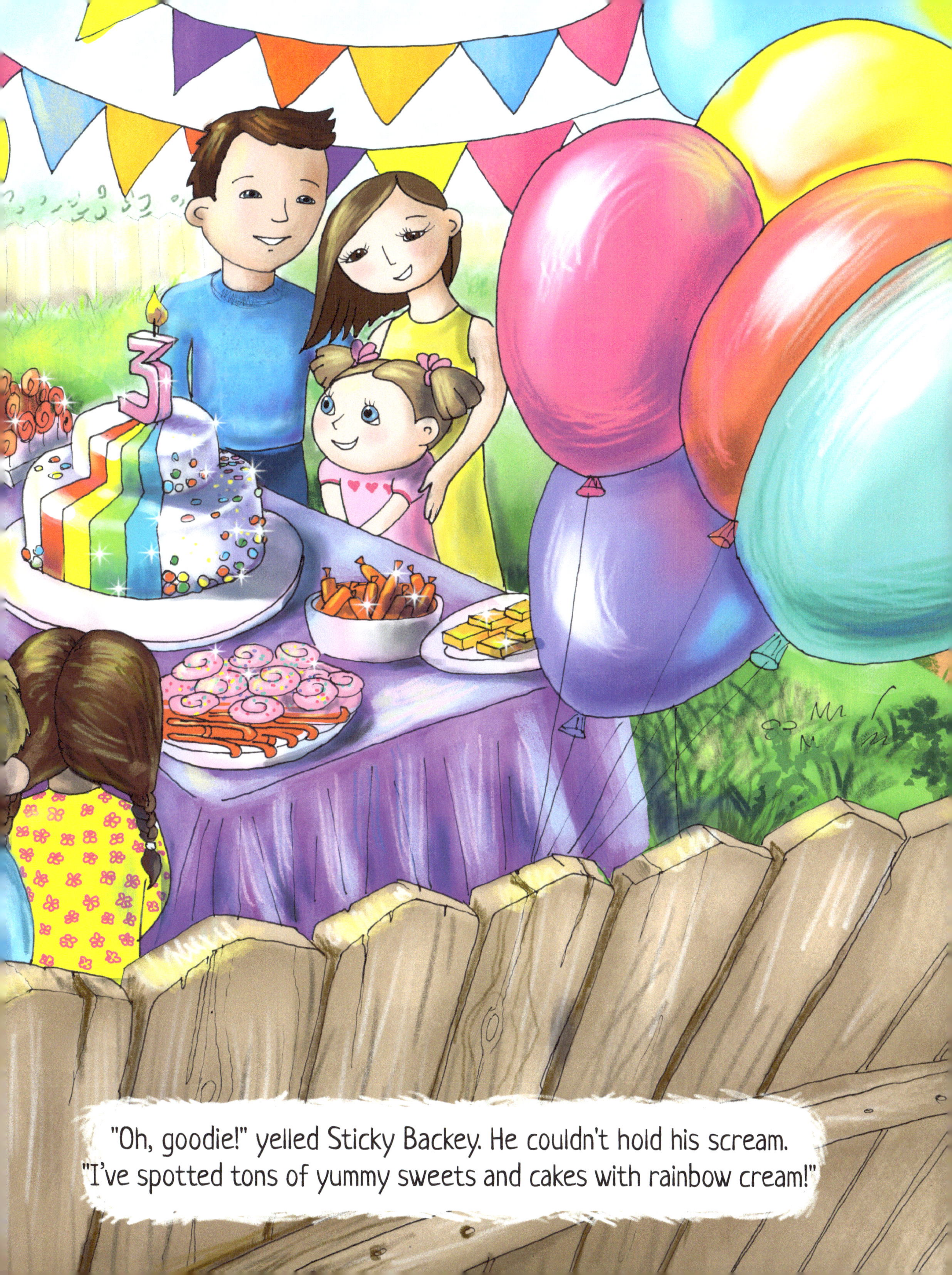
"Oh, goodie!" yelled Sticky Backey. He couldn't hold his scream.
"I've spotted tons of yummy sweets and cakes with rainbow cream!"

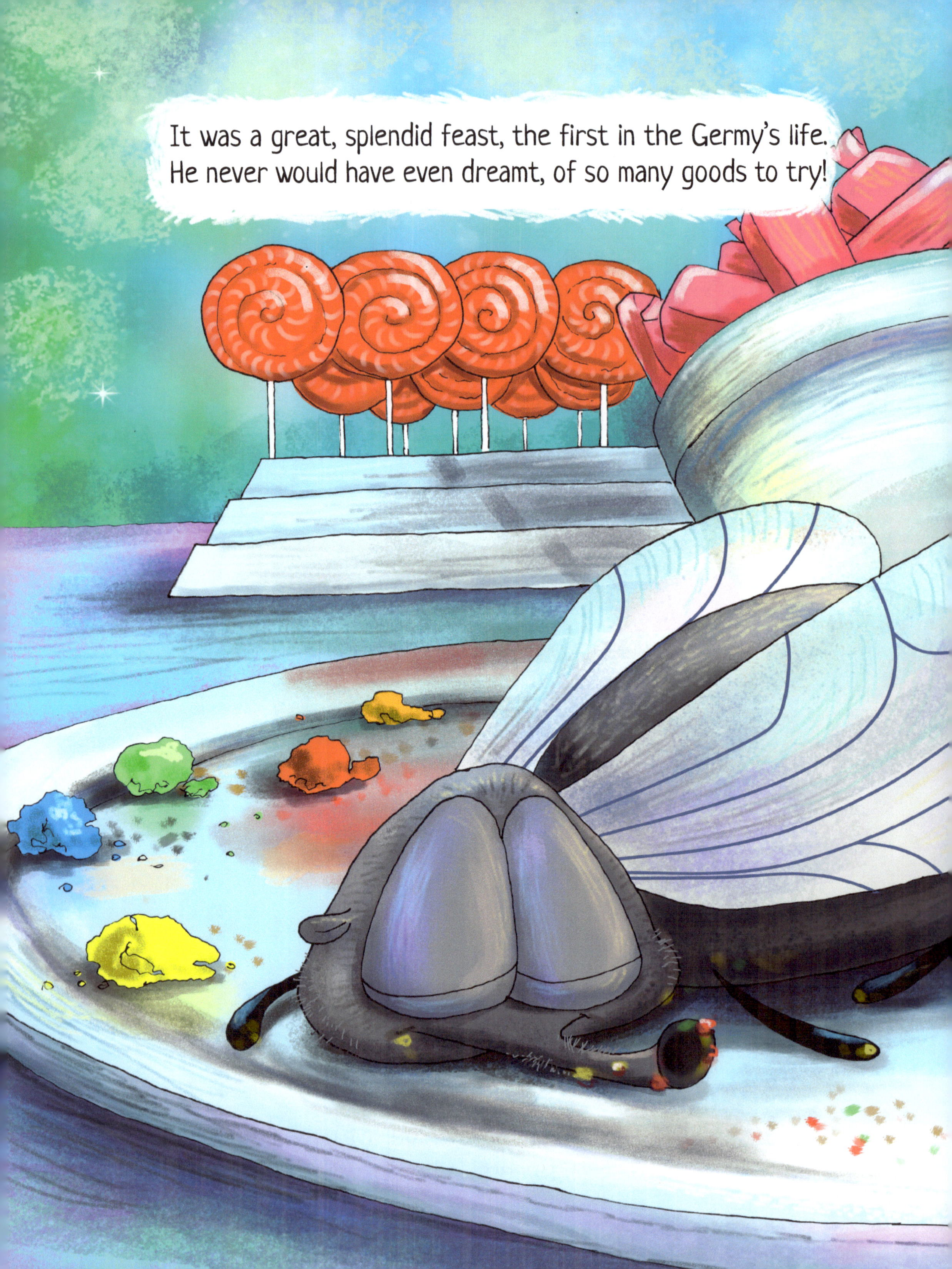
It was a great, splendid feast, the first in the Germy's life.
He never would have even dreamt, of so many goods to try!

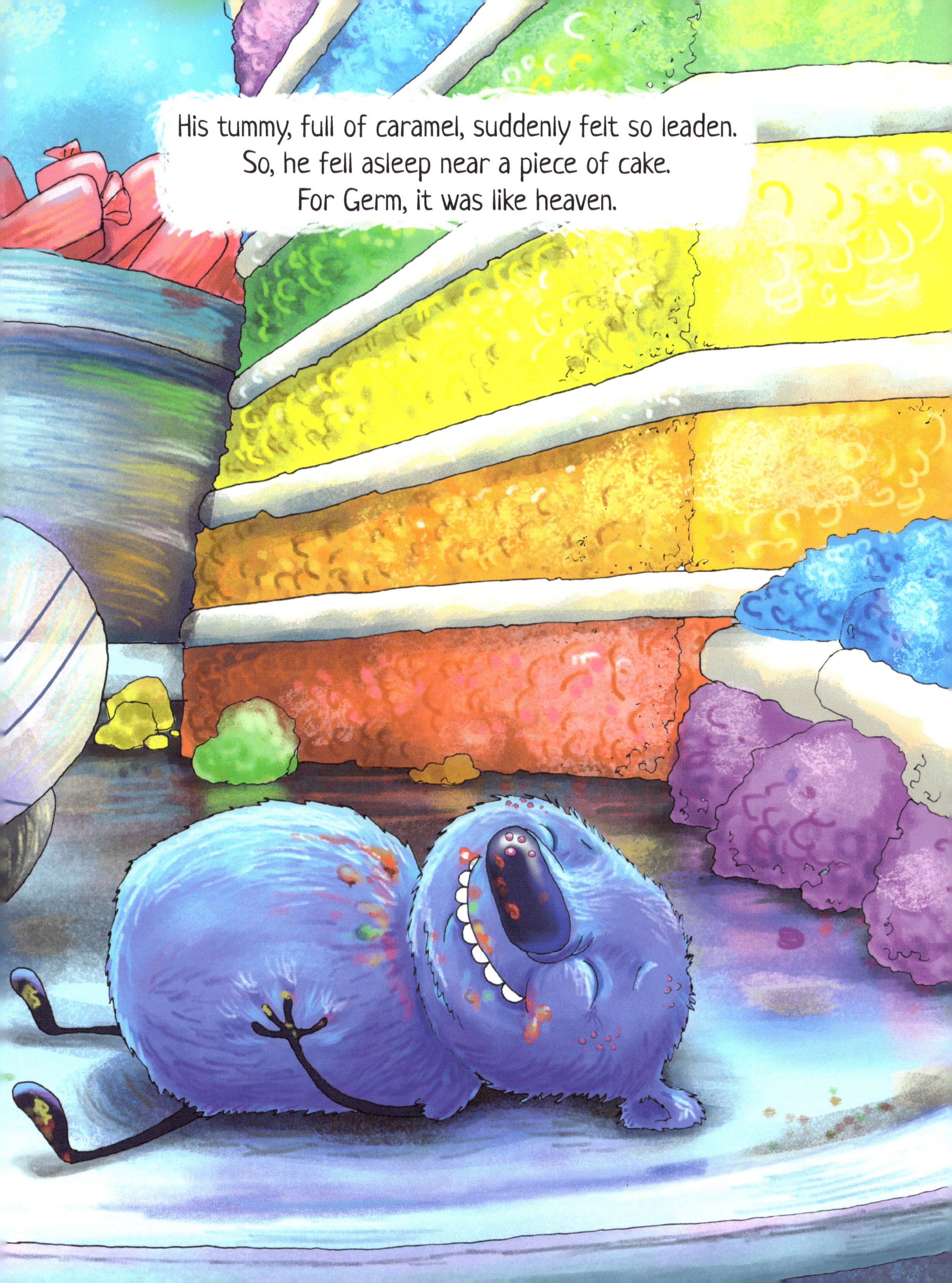
His tummy, full of caramel, suddenly felt so leaden.
So, he fell asleep near a piece of cake.
For Germ, it was like heaven.

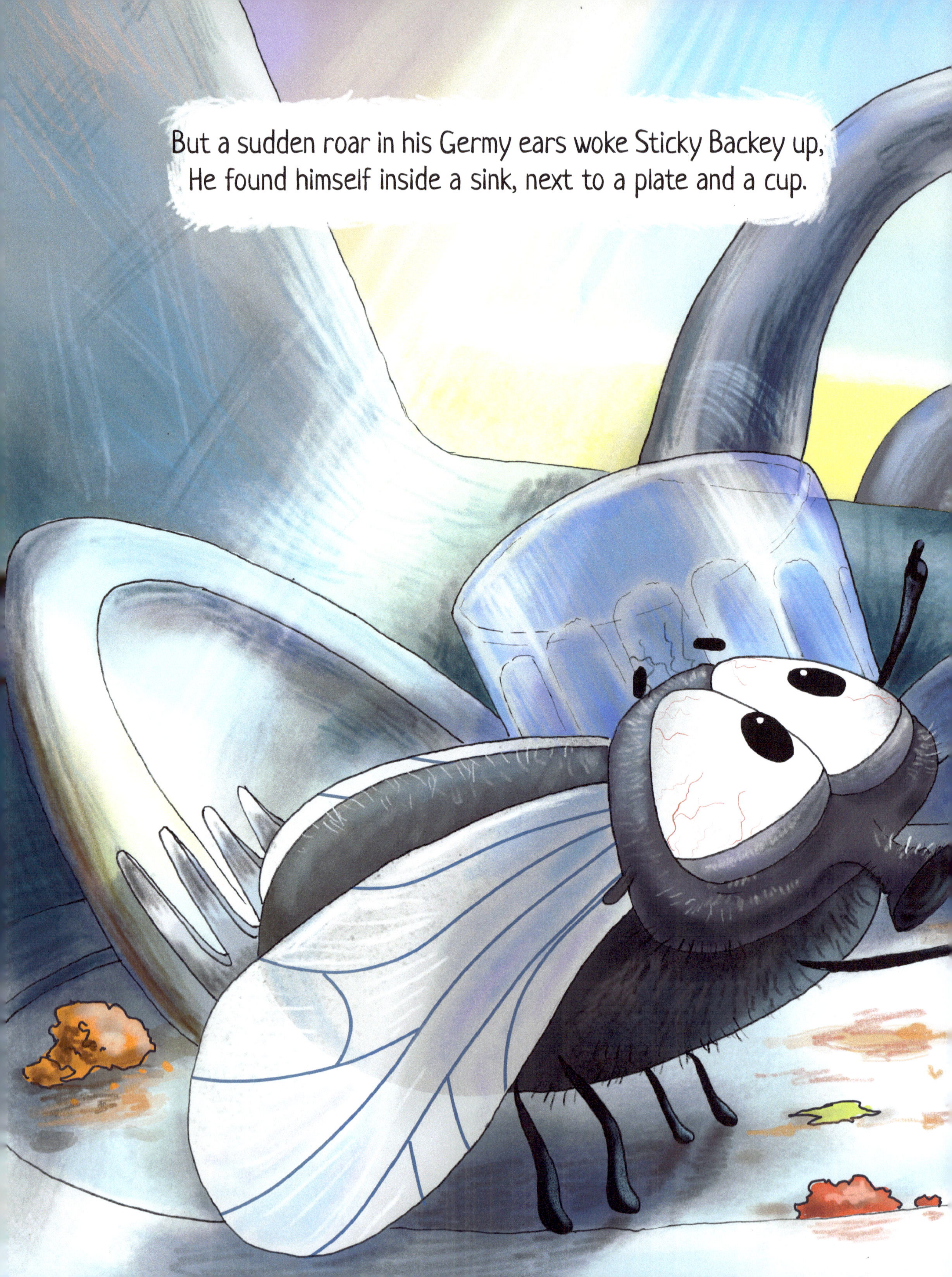
But a sudden roar in his Germy ears woke Sticky Backey up,
He found himself inside a sink, next to a plate and a cup.

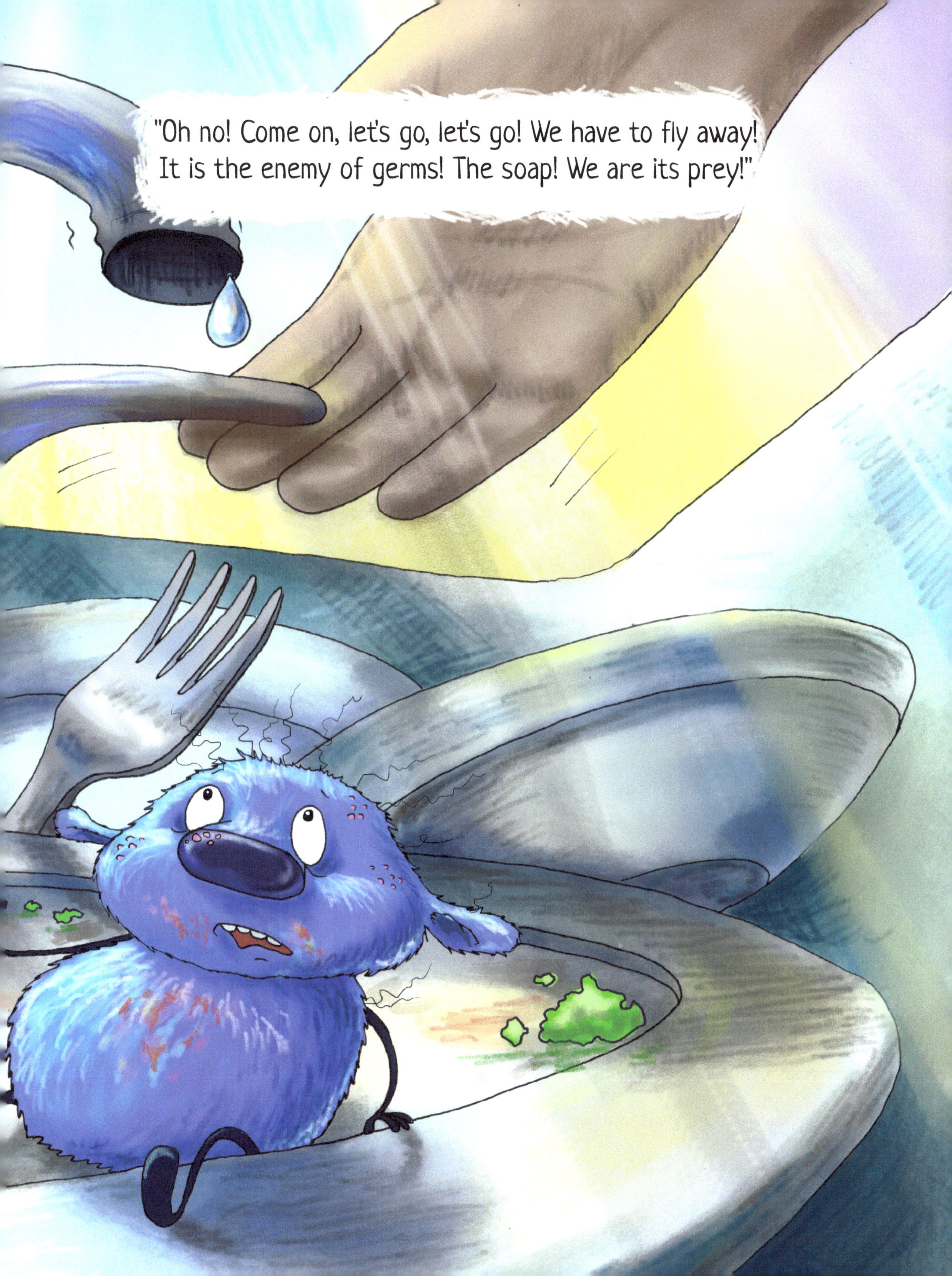

"Oh no! Come on, let's go, let's go! We have to fly away! It is the enemy of germs! The soap! We are its prey!"

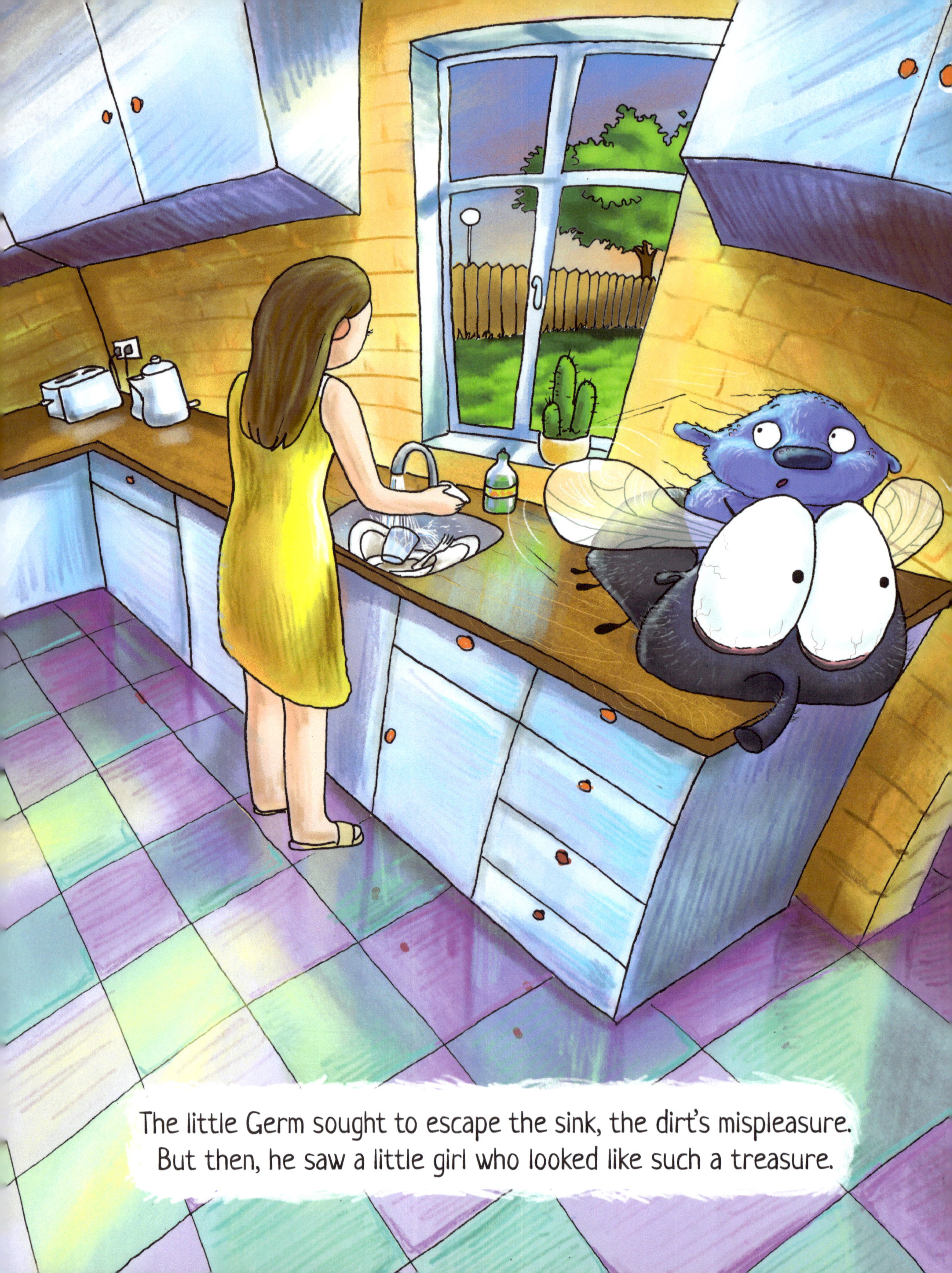

The little Germ sought to escape the sink, the dirt's mispleasure.
But then, he saw a little girl who looked like such a treasure.

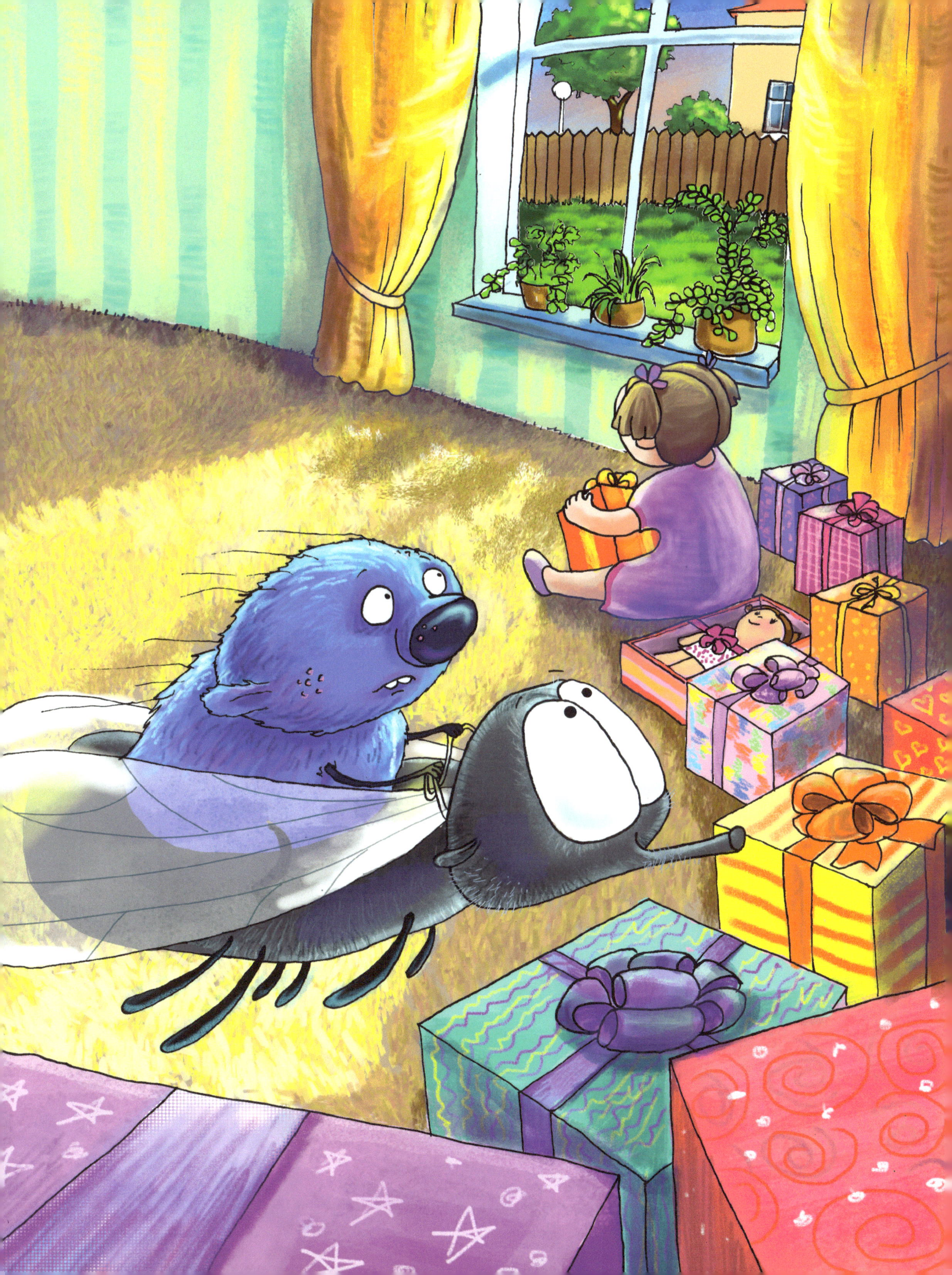

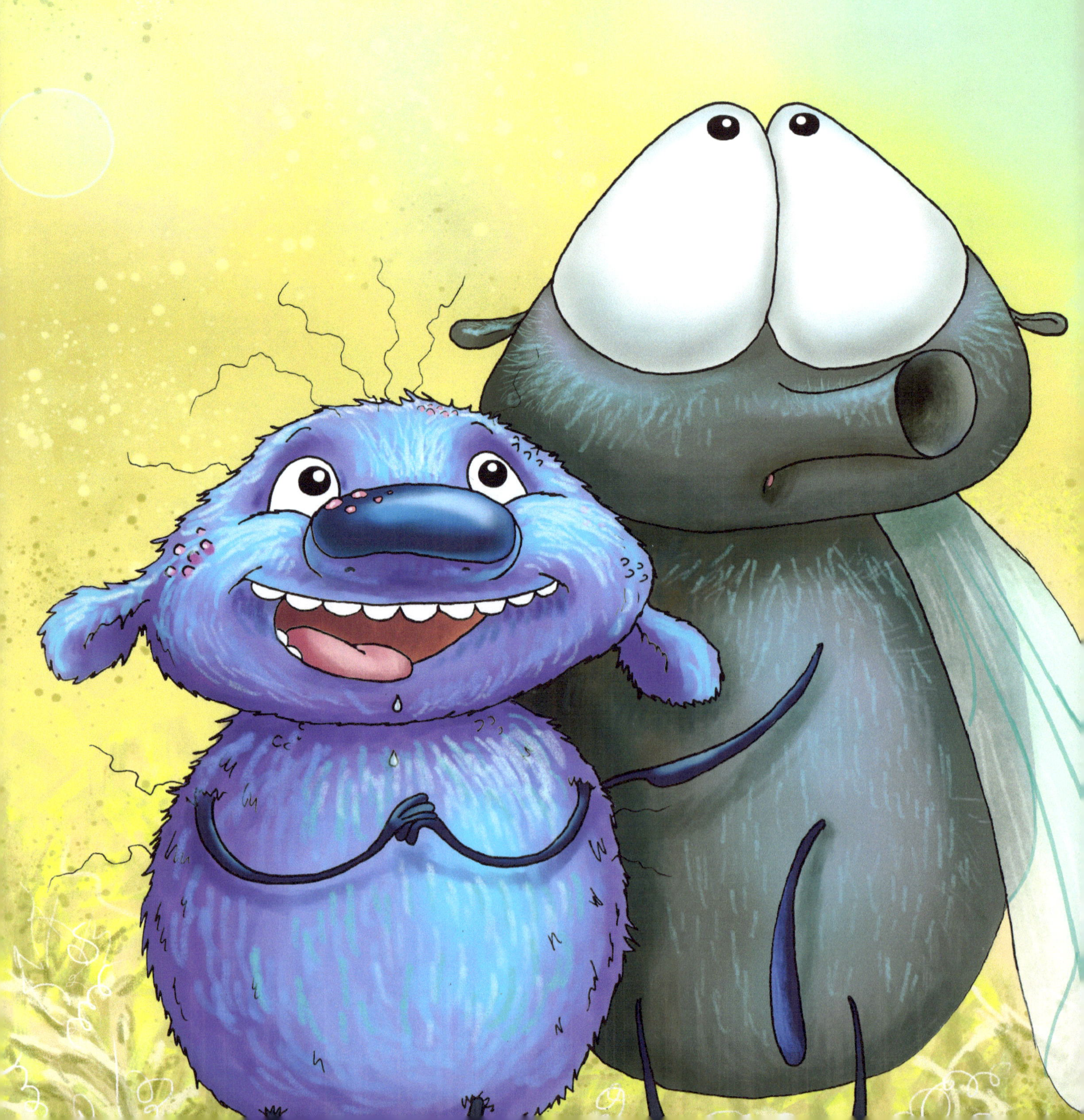
"Oh, what a miracle, that kid! Her face so sweet and greasy,
Her dress is all covered in stains! Just perfect, nothing's missing!

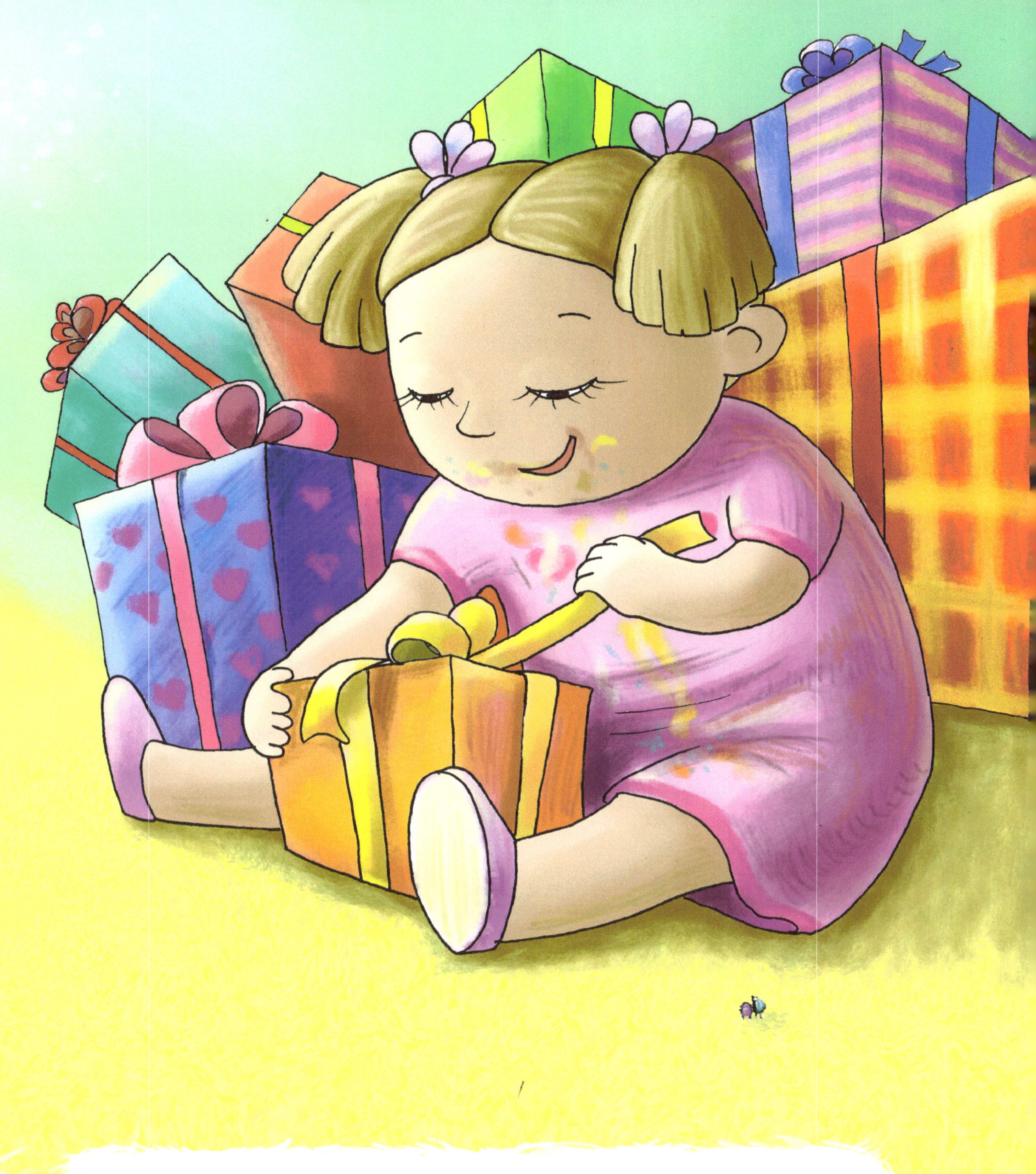

I can see our future dirty life, we were made to be together!
And other germs, I'm pretty sure, will be here soon, foregather!"

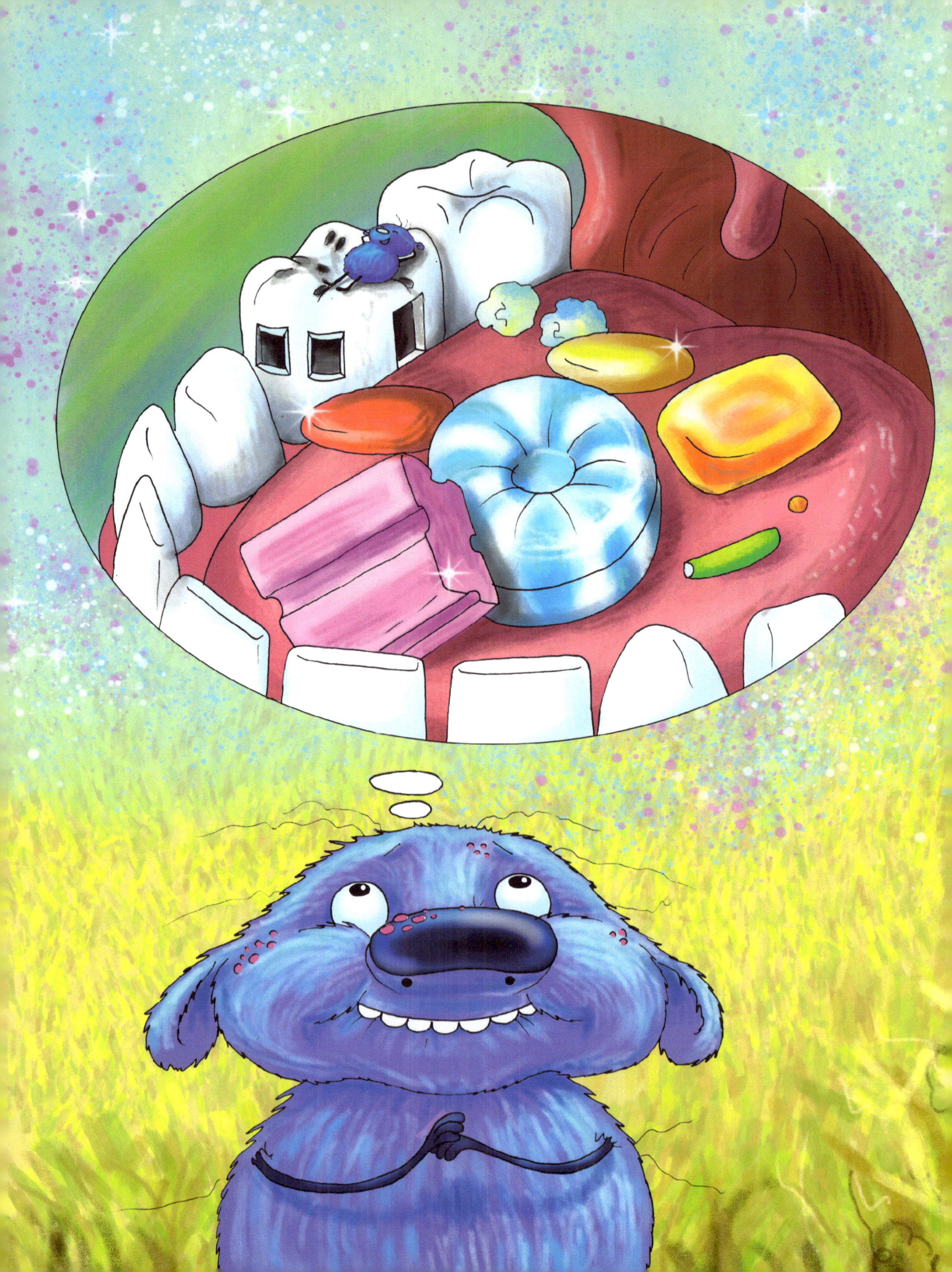

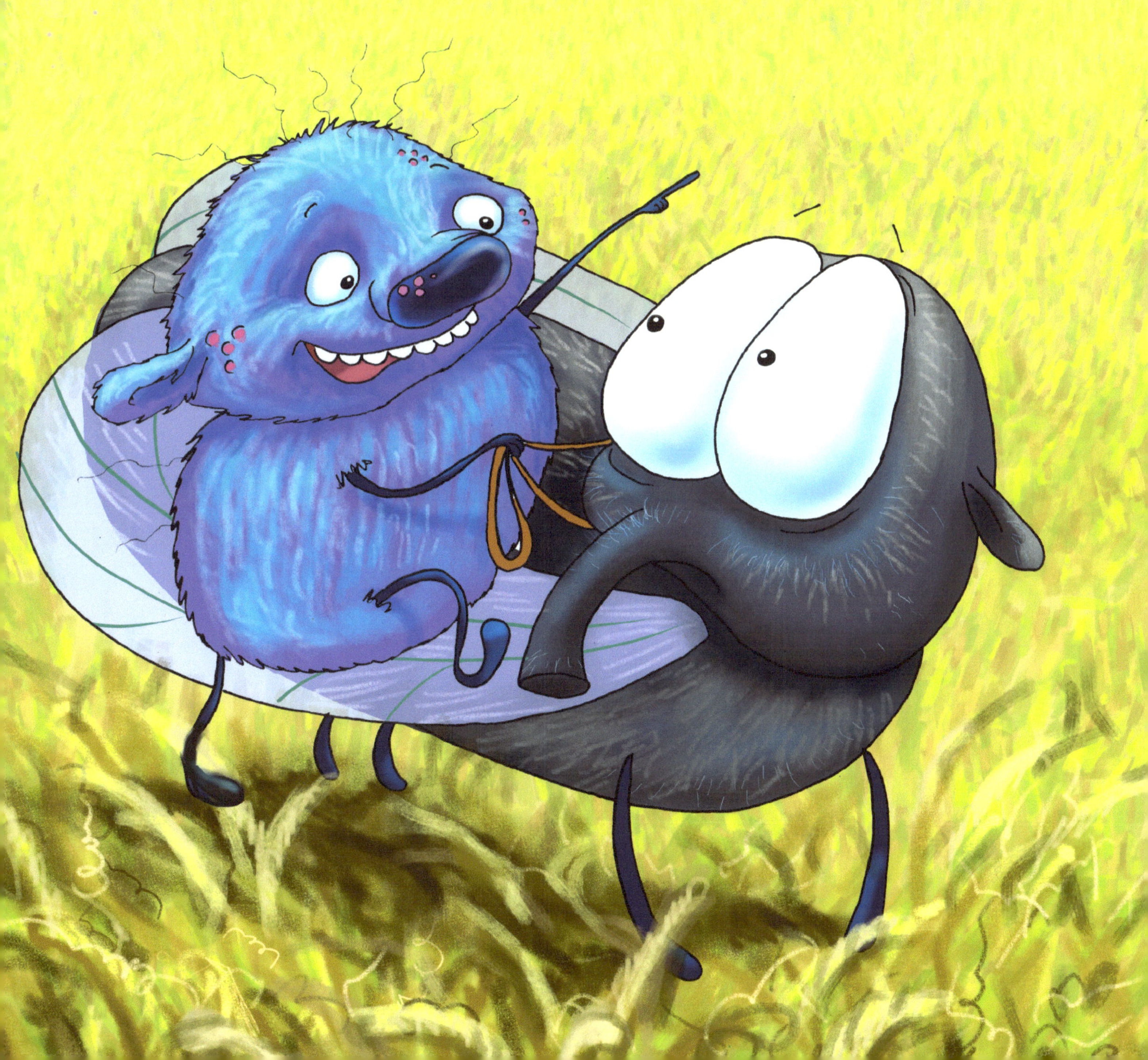
"I am going to build a cozy home in her teeny tiny tooth,
And every day will be so sweet, my life will be so smooth!
Let's all go there, my little friend! My target is her mouth,
And I can't wait to dig a cavity and build my cozy house!"

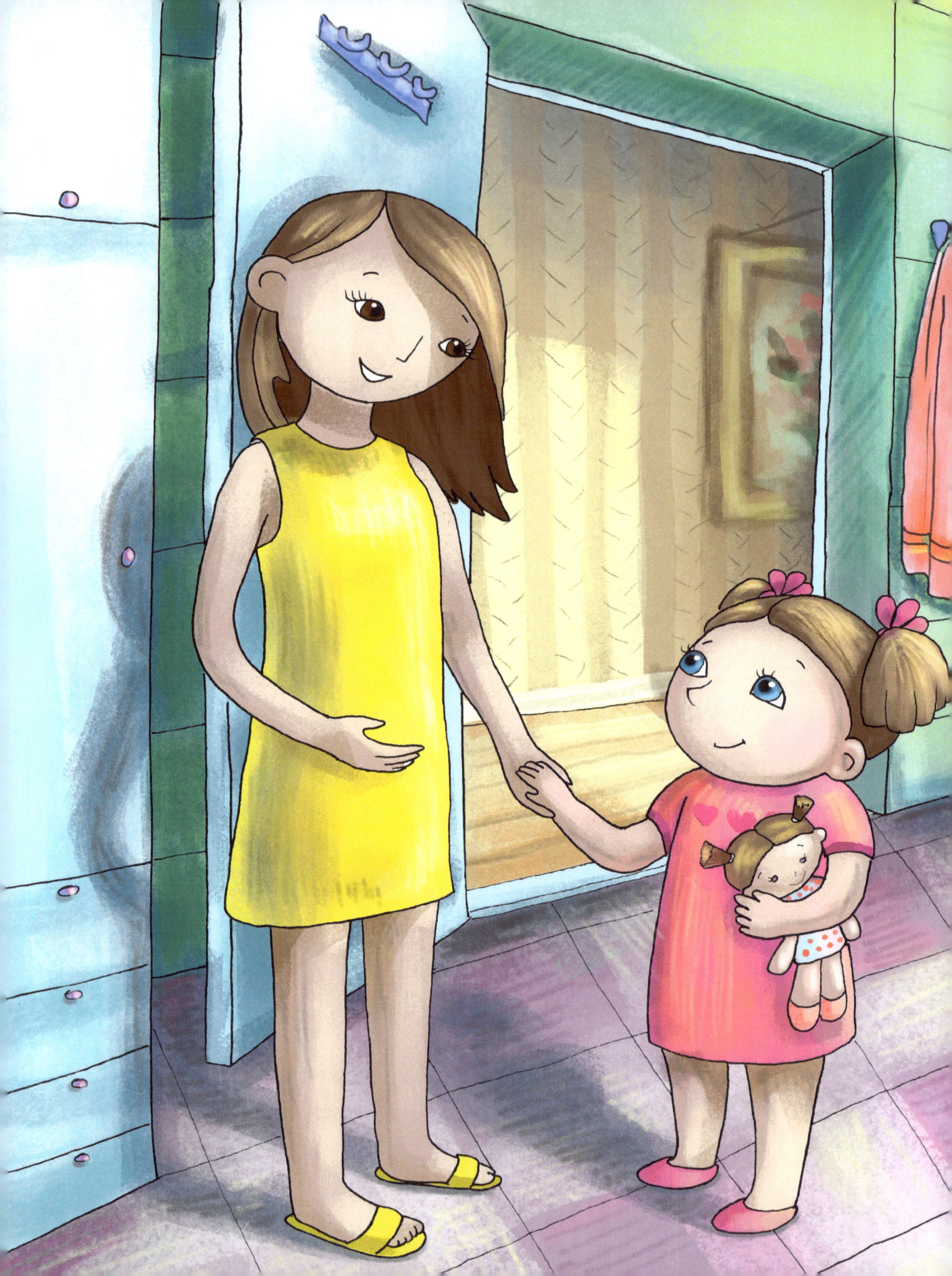

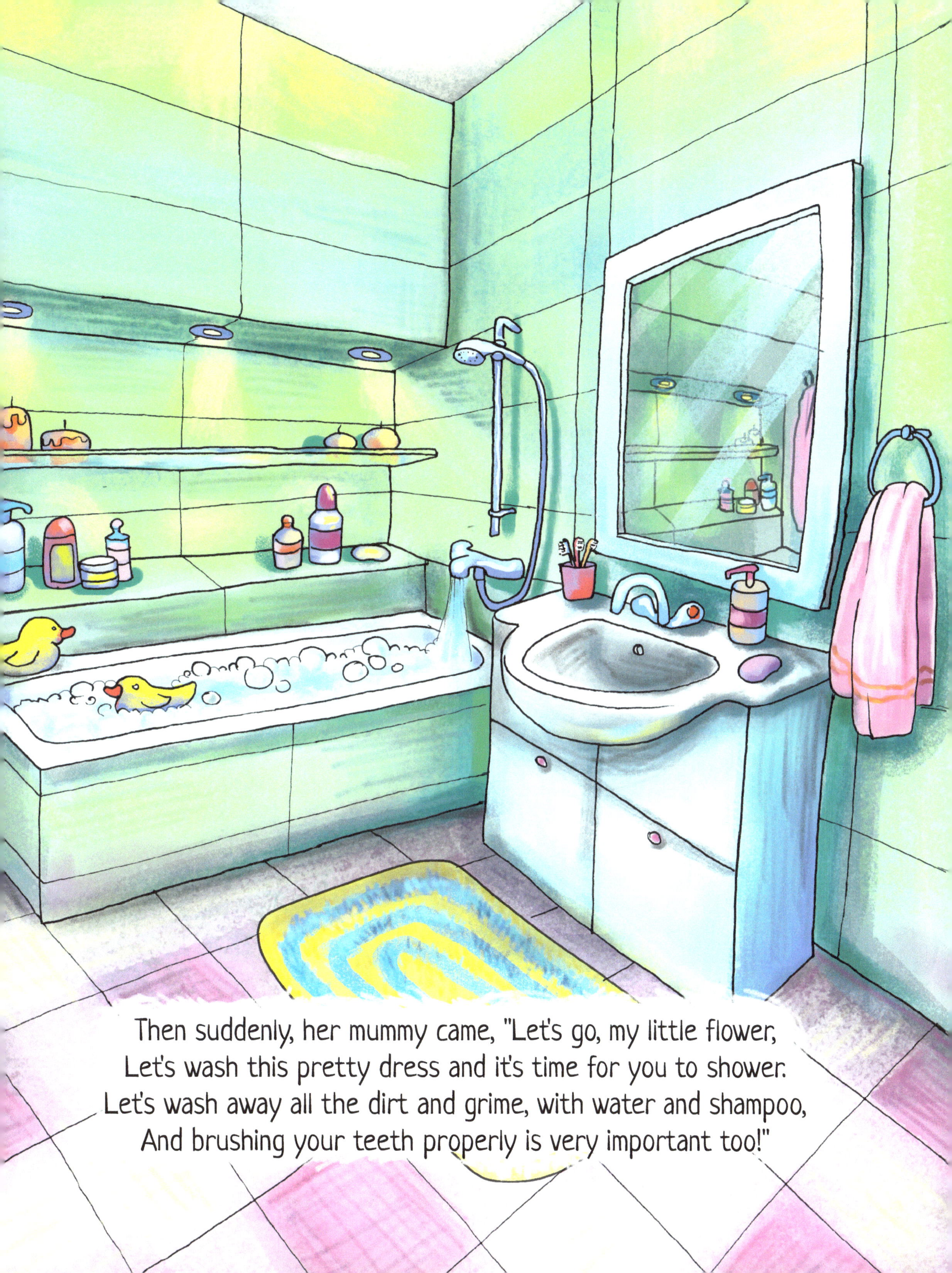

Then suddenly, her mummy came, "Let's go, my little flower,
Let's wash this pretty dress and it's time for you to shower.
Let's wash away all the dirt and grime, with water and shampoo,
And brushing your teeth properly is very important too!"

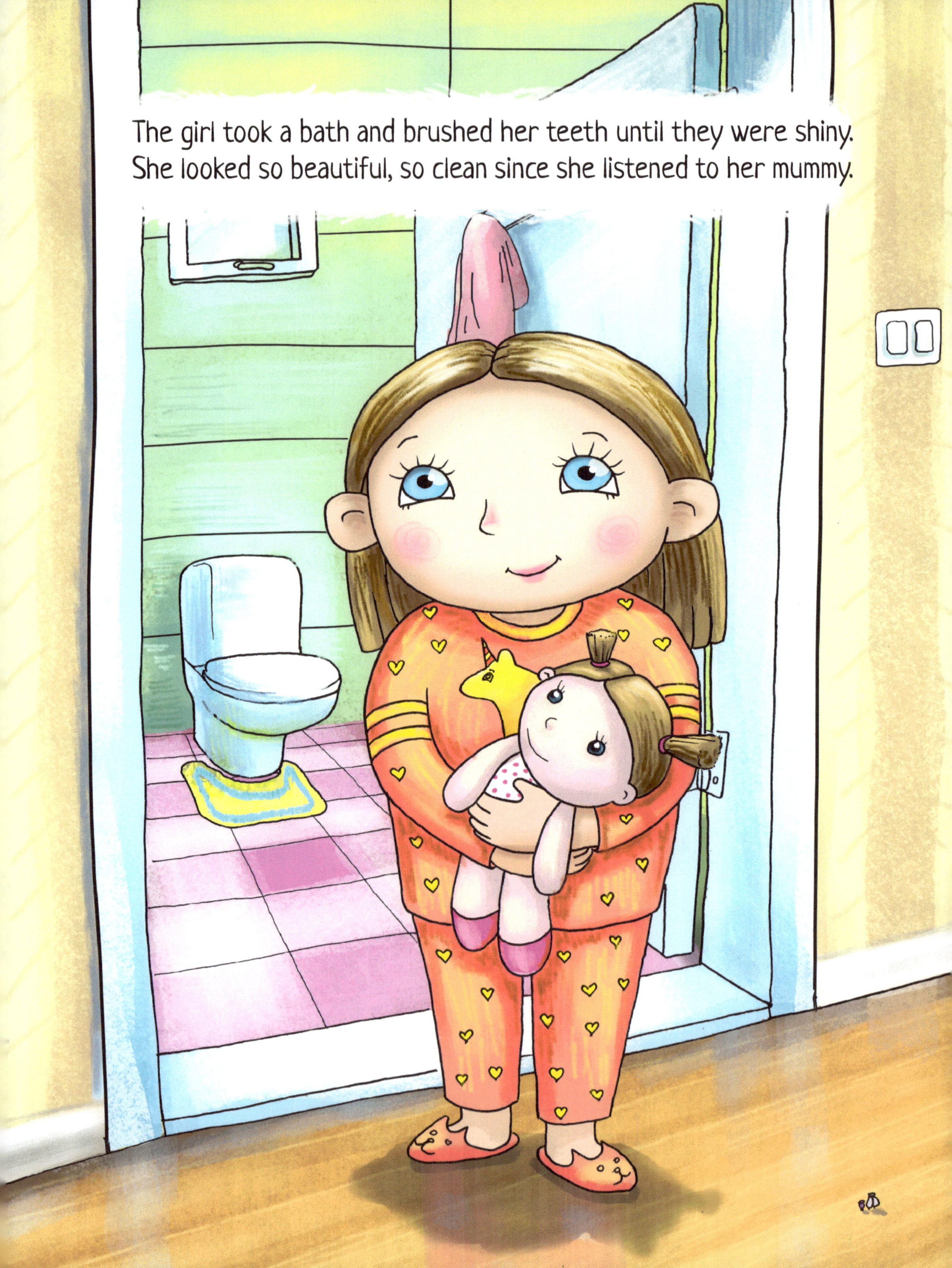

The girl took a bath and brushed her teeth until they were shiny.
She looked so beautiful, so clean since she listened to her mummy.

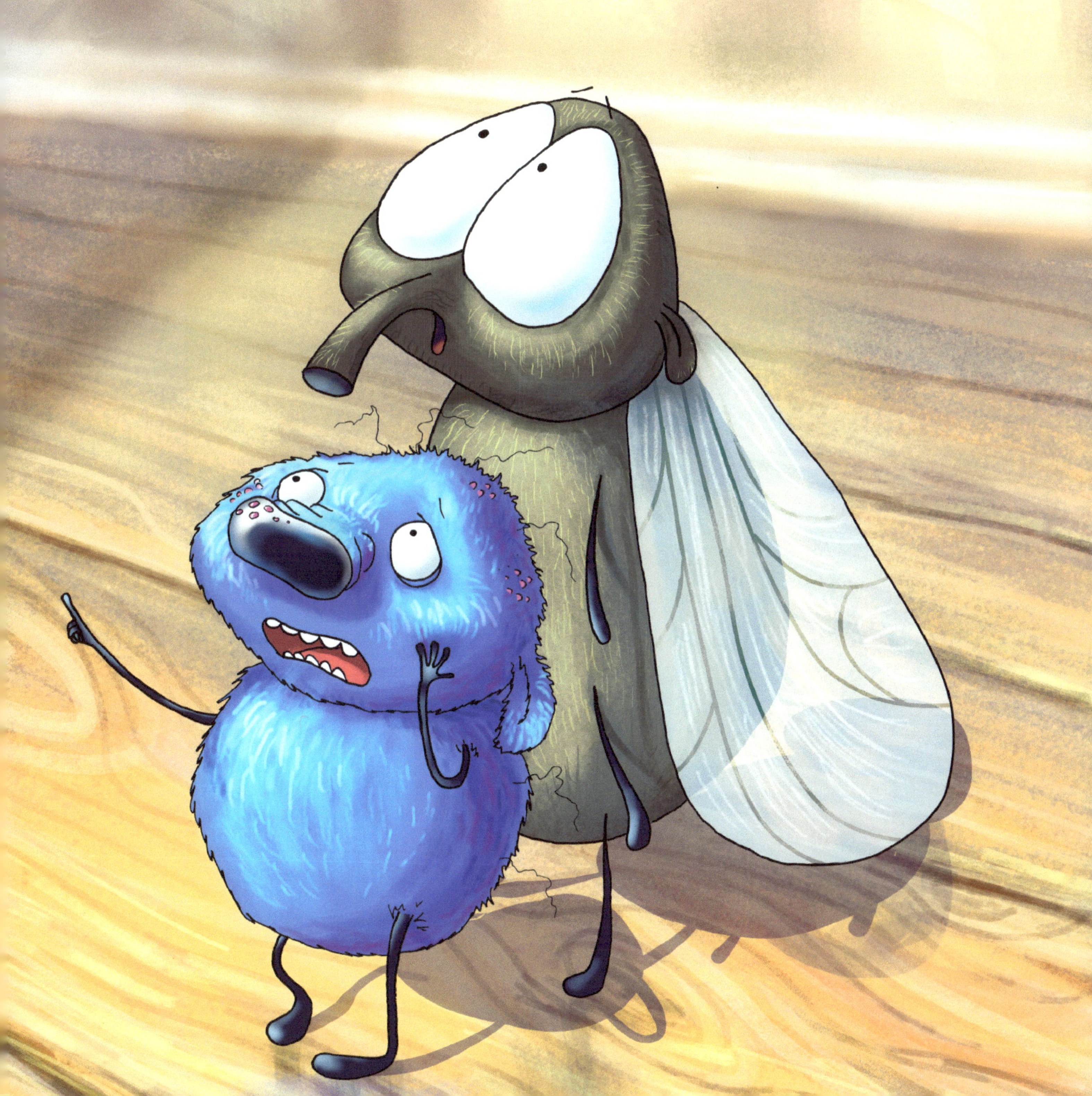

"Oh no! No way! I can't believe!" the little Germy sneered.
"The caramel was in her teeth, and now it's disappeared?
And all that lovely dirt and stains, they have completely vanished.
What's happening? Why is it gone? Why am I being punished?"

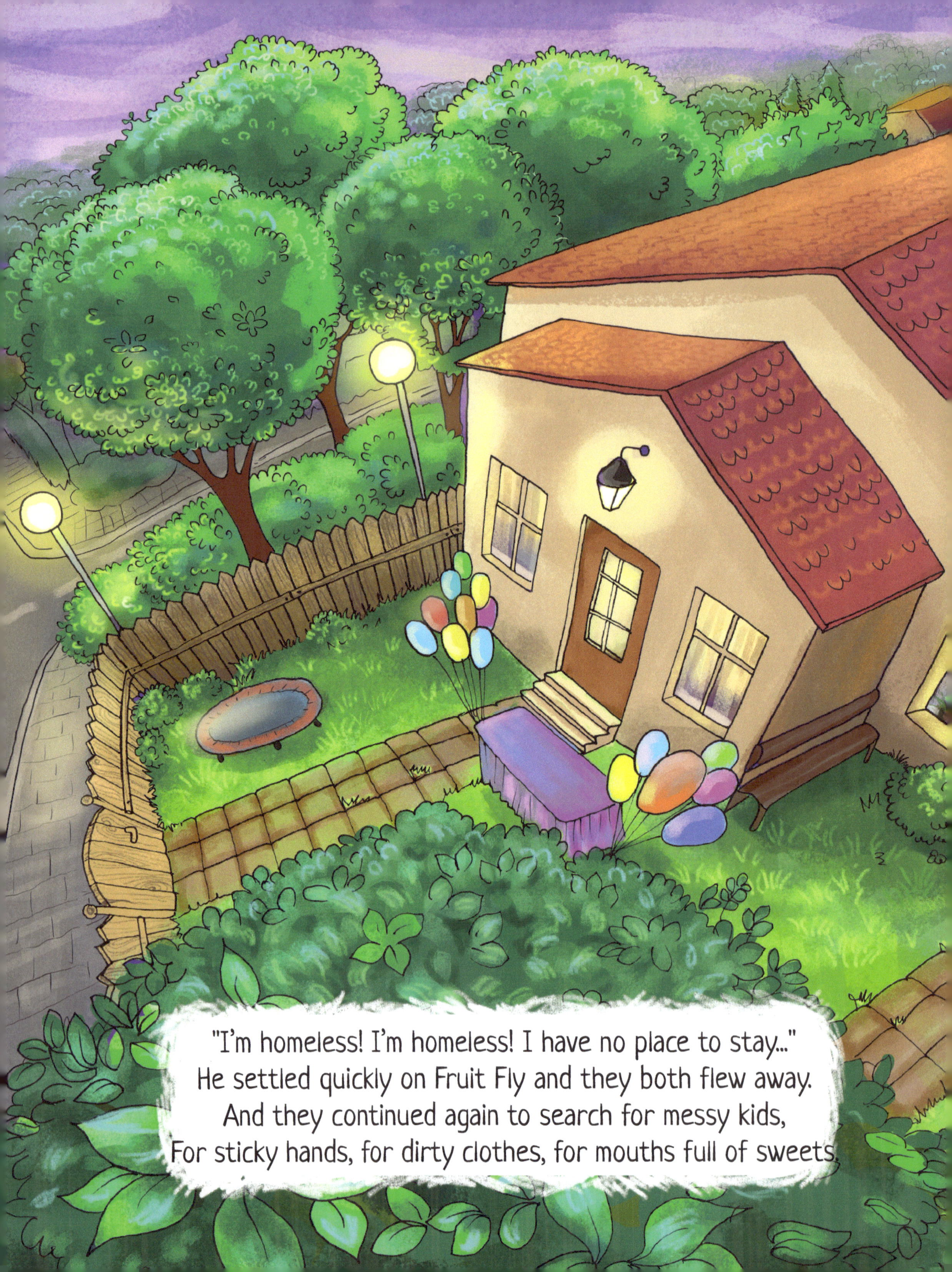

"I'm homeless! I'm homeless! I have no place to stay..."
He settled quickly on Fruit Fly and they both flew away.
And they continued again to search for messy kids,
For sticky hands, for dirty clothes, for mouths full of sweets.

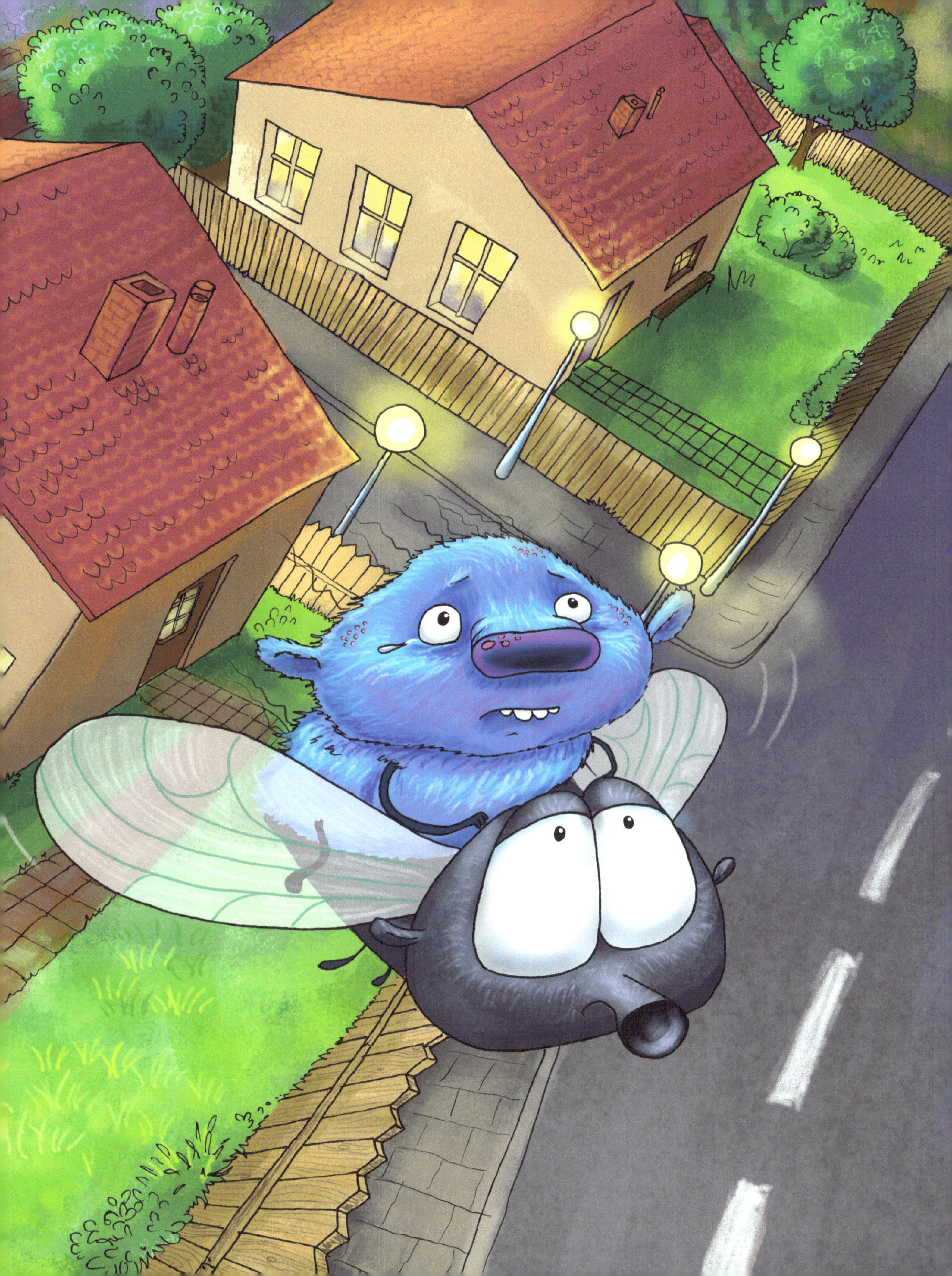

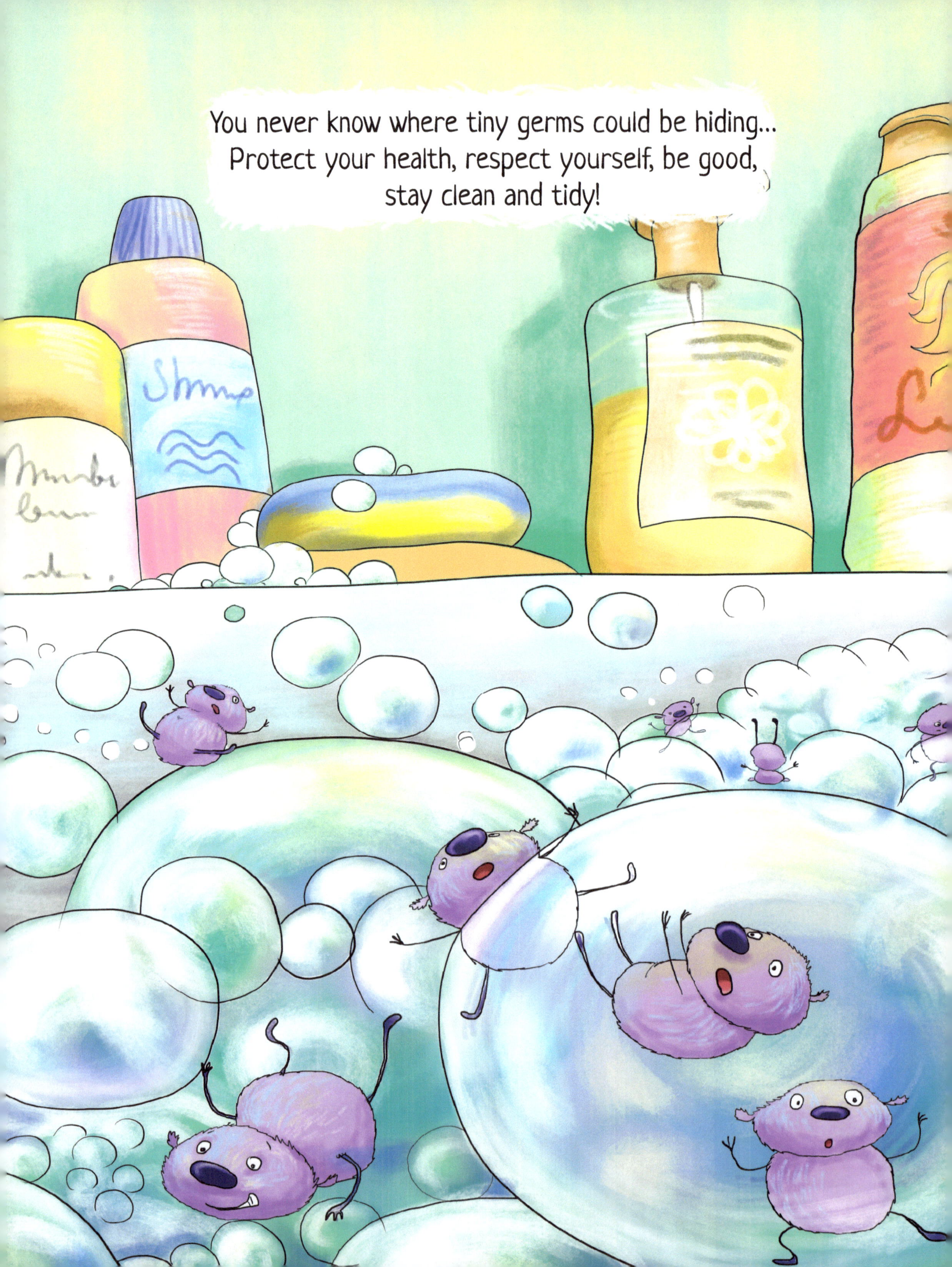

You never know where tiny germs could be hiding...
Protect your health, respect yourself, be good,
stay clean and tidy!

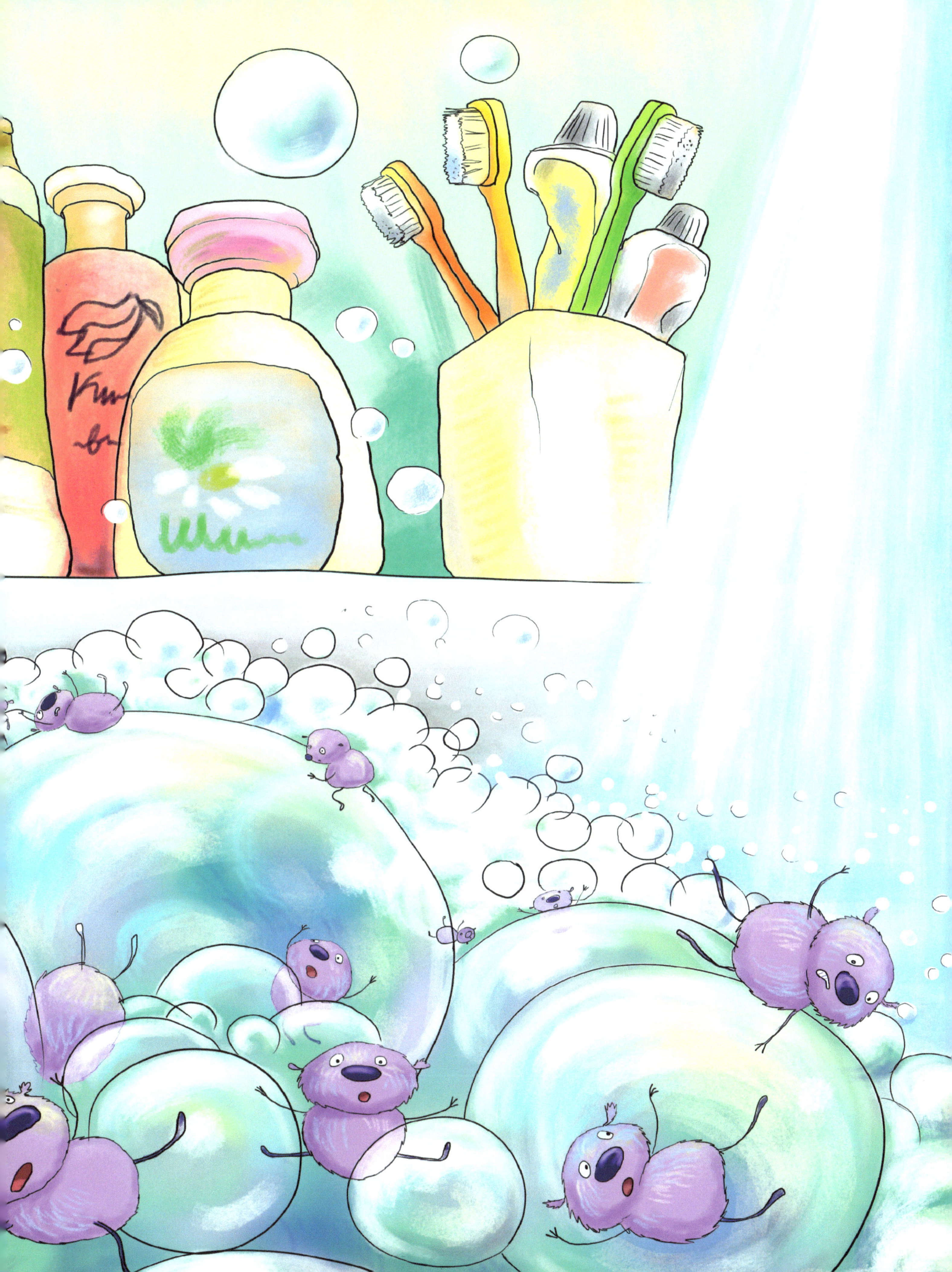

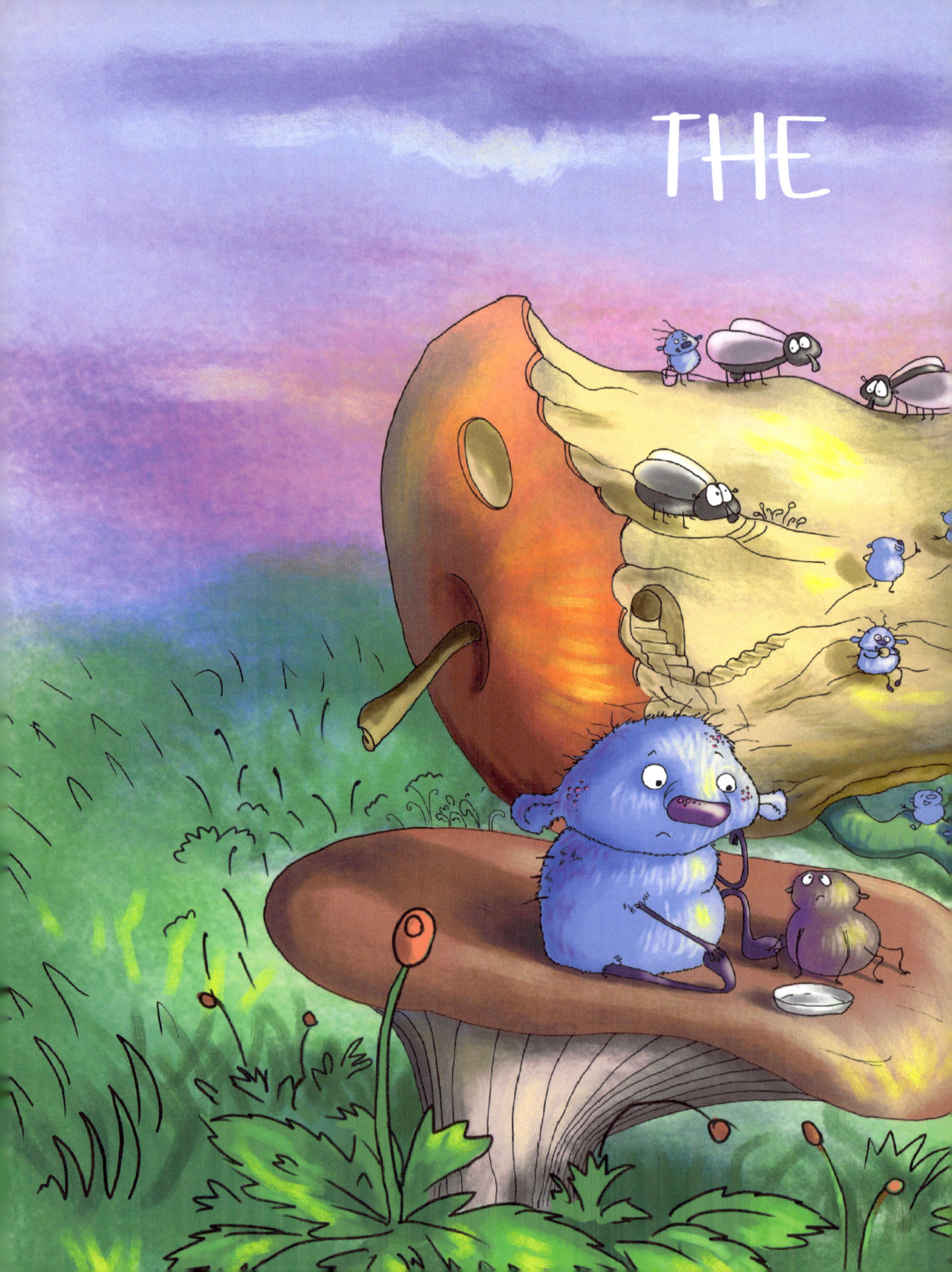
THE

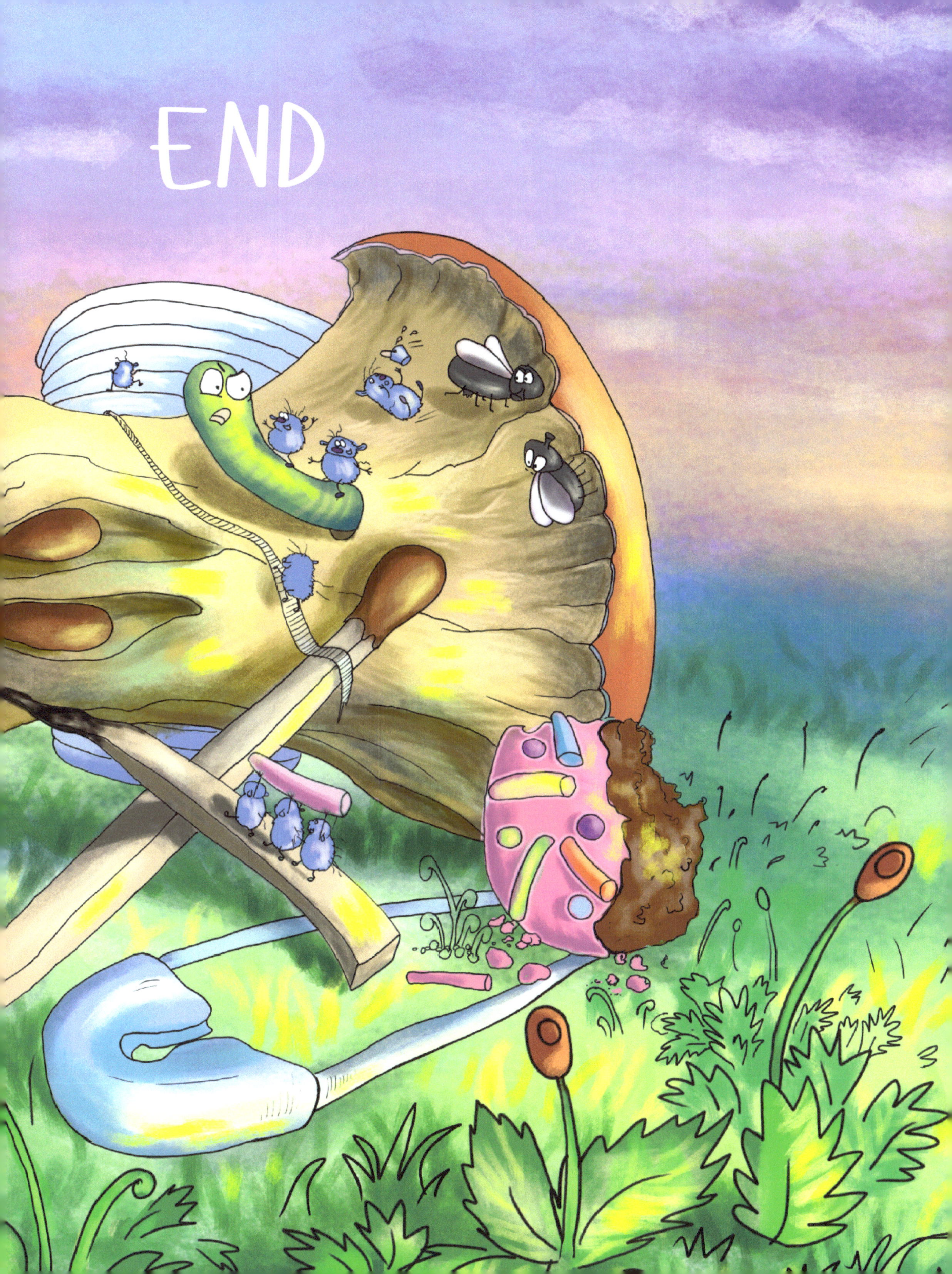

END

# STICKY BACKEY

Written and illustrated by

## Viktoriia Oliinyk

Edited by

## Emily Abdelmegid